HAWAIIAN HERBS
OF MEDICINAL VALUE

TERRITORIAL BOARD OF HEALTH

HAWAIIAN HERBS

OF MEDICINAL VALUE

Found Among the Mountains and Elsewhere
in the Hawaiian Islands, and Known to
the Hawaiians to Possess Curative
and Palliative Properties
Most Effective in Removing Physical Ailments

Translated by AKAIKO AKANA, from the
Original Compilations of Messrs. D. M. Kaaiakamanu and J. K. Akina,
Employees of the Board of Health of the Territory of Hawaii

Classification of Herbs made by H. F. BERGMAN, Ph. D.
Prof. of Botany University of Hawaii

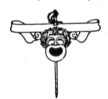

A FACSIMILE REPRINT

PACIFIC BOOK HOUSE
Honolulu, Hawaii

CHARLES E. TUTTLE COMPANY
Rutland, Vermont & Tokyo, Japan

NOTE

HAWAIIAN HERBS OF MEDICINAL VALUE was first published in 1922. Since the original publication is long out of print and is extremely scarce, we are undertaking this reprint in the interest of cultural research. Neither we nor the Hawaii State Department of Health, who so kindly gave us permission to reprint, endorse or make any claim as to the efficacy of the remedies given. Nor do we guarantee the accuracy of the scientific identifications of the herbs used.

PACIFIC BOOK HOUSE

Library of Congress Catalog Card No. 76-177367
International Standard Book No. 0-8048-1019-2

Printed in Japan

Hawaiian Herbs of Medicinal Value

FOUND AMONG THE MOUNTAINS AND ELSEWHERE IN
THE HAWAIIAN ISLANDS AND KNOWN TO THE
HAWAIIANS TO POSSESS CURATIVE AND
PALLIATIVE PROPERTIES
MOST EFFECTIVE IN REMOVING PHYSICAL AILMENTS

*Translated by Akaiko Akana, from the Original Compila-
tions of Messrs. D. M. Kaaiakamanu and
J. K. Akina, Employees of the
Board of Health of the Territory of Hawaii*

1. **A-A-LI-I (or "KUMAKANI"—"Standing against strong wind or gale.")**
   (*Dodonaea viscosa*)

This is a low-growing plant. It is hard and stiff, thus enabling it to resist the Kona-gale. It is found at the edge of cliffs among the mountains of Hawaii. Because of its power to resist the Kona-gale, it is named "ku-makani."

Its leaves are full, something like the "lehua" leaf, and are invaluable because of its power to destroy rash and itch.

In preparing it, take a medium-size container and fill it with the leaves of the "A-a-li-i." Add eight pieces of "puakala-ku-kula" (no scientific name), tap-root bark together with the bark of A-la-a (*Sderoxylon*)—the portion that touches the ground. Pound these until thoroughly mixed and then empty the mixture into another container. Add to this sufficient amount of water, at the same time throwing in four pickings (taking with thumb and fore-finger) of salt. Mix the contents thoroughly and then clean by allowing the liquid pressed out from the bulk to pass through the finely prepared fibers of the "ahu-awa" (*Cyperus laevigata*). This done, sink four red-hot stones into the liquid. When it steams, cover the container with "kapa" cloth and allow the content to cook. As the liquid cools down to the right temperature, bathe the body with it and, thereafter, repeat the process morning and evening. This remedy is very effective in destroying contagious diseases and in keeping away evil influences. At the close of the application clean the bowels by taking four "pilikai" (*Argreia tiliaefolia*) seeds, ground and reduced to powder form.

This cure is named "holoina" (washed). Hence the old saying: "The affliction being rash or itch, the cure is the "holoina.""

2. **AA-LII MAHU or AA-LII MAKO'I.**
   (Specimen desired for proper identification.)

This herb can be secured at places near the beach, for instance, at Lima-loa, Kauai and Puuhale, Honolulu. The plant is low. Its wood is frequently used for hatchet handles, the kind employed for trimming the end pieces of a canoe, hence the name, "mako-i." The leaves resemble those of the "naio." Its flowers are white and has berries similar to those of the "popolo" (no scientific name given).

Only the two-leaf bud of this herb is used for medicine, and is applied in case of hard cold in the head and headache.

To prepare it, take sixteen buds of the "aa-lii mahu" with two pickings of salt. Rub these between the thumb and forefinger until the juice appears. Then inhale the fume that arises until the nostrils flow. This brings relief.

3. AIEA or HALENA. (Specimen desired for proper identification.)

The wood of this herb is very hard like that of the "ahakea" and is usually employed in making the end pieces of canoes. Its leaves are like those of the mountain apple and the juice from the bark is very bitter.

The ripe leaves, together with the bark and tap-root are employed for the cure of ulcers and scrofulous sores.

To prepare and apply it, take twenty ripe leaves of the "aiea" with two pieces of sufficient size of its bark. Pound these to proper consistency with sufficient amount of water. Then press the juice thus obtained into a container and clean it with the finely prepared fibers of the "ahuawa" (*Cyperus laevigata*). This done, put into the liquid four heated stones to cook it. Then the liquid is allowed to cool. The tapa cloth is then taken and soaked with the medicine and applied on the sores as a wash.

Because of its bitterness, the liquid, in any way, should not be brought in contact with the mouth and eyes.

Since it is necessary to keep the bowels clean while the application is being made, this remedy should be taken: Two pieces of "ohia" (mountain apple) of sufficient size; two pieces of "ohia-lehua" (*Jambosa malaecensia*); two whole bushes of "moa" (*Psilotum triquetrum*); three segments of reddish sugar-cane, pounded together and the juice extracted and cleaned with the finely prepared fibers of the "ahuawa" (*Cyperus laevigata*) and taken internally in equal amounts morning and evening for five consecutive days.

4. AU-A-INA. (Specimen desired for proper identification.)

The bark of this herb is rough and hard. It is very difficult to find it owing to its scarcity. It may be found on the slopes of the Kona side of Mauna Loa and in the neighborhood of Waimanu, Hawaii; also at Nahiku and towards the mountain at Kipahulu and Kaupo on Maui. It grows on the Kahana mountains, Oahu; also on Limahuli, Kauai.

The part used for medicine is the wood of the herb. It is first dried and then scraped with the "opihi" shell. The scraping is chewed with dried cocoanut-meat and swallowed. The "oo" leaves of sufficient quantity are then taken and soaked in water over night with eight pieces of *Waltheria americana* tap-root bark and two segments of white sugar-cane. These are pounded together thoroughly and the juice cleansed by being pressed through the finely prepared fibers of the *Cyperus laevigata*. The liquid, in a pint-size container, is taken internally three times a day for five successive days. This remedy, or treatment, is largely used for cleansing the blood and for stimulating the appetite. In some cases, it is applied like the *Dodonaea ciscosa* and *Sideroxylon*.

5. AU-HU-HU. (*Tephrosia piscatoria*)

This herb grows on cliffs, in valleys and on hill-sides. It is a low-growing plant with leaves like those of the *Sida* spp., having yellowish white flowers. The herb is poisonous.

This remedy is employed for skin diseases like rash, itch, scales, ulcers, etc. To prepare it, take forty young leaves or buds, add about a tablespoonful of Hawaiian salt and with baked (over charcoal) piece of cocoanut and sufficient amount of water mixed with a sufficient amount of a child's urine, are pounded to proper consistency. The liquid thus secured is cleansed by pressing it through finely prepared cocoanut fibers. The preparation is then ready for application. Not only is it beneficial to the skin but to deep cuts as well.

This medicine should not be given to children. Because it is used for poisoning fish, it is called "hola," or "au-hola."

6. AU-KO-I or PI HOHONO or MIKIPALAOA. (*Cassis occidentalis*)

This herb does not grow very high. Its leaves are oblong, having yellowish flowers and bearing pods.

As a remedy, it is largely employed for the cure of skin troubles like ring-worm, white blotches of the skin and other similar diseases. In pre-

paring it, take the entire plant from leaf to root, eliminating the seeds.
Add about a tablespoonful of salt, one "opihi"-shell, four "haukeuke" shells,
(covers of dark purple sea-egg that clings to the rocks by means of tiny
suckers, and moving by means of paddle-like prongs having dull points); a
sufficient amount of child urine; papaia milk and the juice of kukui-nuts
(the juice of the young nuts that comes out from where they break off from
the stems). Pound these together until thoroughly mixed. Then wrap the
mixture in finely prepared cocoanut fibers and squeeze out the juice. The
liquid thus obtained is then taken and applied on the afflicted parts of the
skin three times a day for five days in succession. As a bath for certain
skin diseases, the entire plant is taken and pounded with water. Then four
heated stones are sunk into the liquid in order to cook it. After it is cooled,
the afflicted parts of the skin are bathed and washed.

As a laxative for cleaning the bowels, "kowali" (*Impomea disectar*) is
taken. This is followed by the regular drinking of the "kookoolau" (*Campylotheca* spp.) tea in order to strengthen the body tissues.

7. AHAKEA. (*Bobea* spp.)

Ahakea is plentiful among the mountains of the Hawaiian Islands. It
grows to an enormous size. Its bark, which is very thick, is bitter, and this
is part of the tree that is used for remedy. Its wood is frequently used for
canoe making or for any of its parts.

The bark is used for blood purifying or for the cure of ulcers. In preparing it, take six pieces of the "ahakea" bark the size of the palm of the
hand, eight pieces of "puakala" tap-root bark, four pieces of the mountain
apple bark and eight *Cassis occidentalis* roots.

These are pounded thoroughly. The mixture is then placed on a banana
leaf and wrapped for stock supply. In case of ulcer, take sufficient amount
of the mixture to produce a handful of the juice. This is placed in finely
prepared cocoanut fibers and through them the juice of the mixture is
squeezed out and put on the afflicted part of the body. This is done twice
a day—morning and evening. But before making the application wash the
sore with a mixture of water and cocoanut milk.

As a blood purifier, take the same mixture and add to it the following:
One cocoanut thoroughly cooked over charcoal, one segment of white sugar
cane, two half-ripe fruits of the *Morinda citrifolia*. These are thoroughly
pounded together and mixed; and, through the finely combed fibers of the
Cyperus laevigata, the juice is pressed out and cleaned and made ready for
use. Then take about a glassful of the liquid before meals. This is immediately followed by an equal amount of water. This is taken twice a day—
morning and evening. Should it be taken as a regular treatment, then the
mixture should have an equal amount of water before being taken. Salty
substances should not be eaten while the treatment is on. Broiled fish and
food cooked with heated stones are very good. Potato and its young leaves,
the "popolo," the young "pakapakai" and "luau" are to be taken. Very
sour poi should not be eaten.

8. AHEWAHEWA. (Specimen desired for proper identification.)

The leaves of the plant are very much like those of the hibiscus and so
are the flowers. The base of the flower is used for stomach trouble, the kind
that whitens the tongue. It is good both for adults and children.

For children from ten to fifty days old, use four flowers (only the base
of the flowers). For those from sixty to eighty days, use a little more than
four, and from that time on to one year the number of flowers correspondingly increases to twelve. This remedy is an easy laxative for the digestive
system, and it should be taken until the bowels move freely.

9. AINA-KEA or KO-KEA. (No specimen.)

This is white sugar cane grown extensively in Hawaii by the natives.
It is whitish green, soft, and very sweet. It is largely used for medical purposes especially in the combination of different herbs. Its special use, how-

ever, is that of relieving the pain and curing internal troubles of the male sexual organ.

In preparing, take four segments of the cane with a whole fully matured cocoanut that is not dried up. Pound these together thoroughly. Then take the mixture and squeeze the juice out through finely prepared cocoanut fibers. The clean liquid is then mixed with about a tablespoonful of the *Hibiscus tiliaceus* juice. This mixture is then dripped into the opening of the male-organ and allowed to flow in as far as possible, thus covering the afflicted region or regions. The treatment is applied three times a day—before and after the passage of water each time. Drink abundance of spring water or the milk of young cocoanut. Do not use salty food or sour poi. Broiled fish or fish cooked in "ti" leaves, "luau" (young taro leaf), "kukui" nut, potatoes and bananas are good articles of food to consume. Take *Ipomea dissecta* for laxative for cleaning the bowels.

10. AHIHI (KU MAKUA). (No specimen for identification.)

This tree resembles the "lehua" in growth and flowers. Its leaves are similar to those of the big-leaf "maile." It may be found at Kilohana, Kalihi-uka, and up towards Waiakeakue and Manoa mountains; also at Keanae and Iao Valley, Maui. It may be found among the mountains of Hawaii and Kauai.

This remedy is useful for cold—the stuffed-up condition of the nostrils, headache and eye-ache, chills, and pains at joints. The application, however, is not the same in all cases.

For stuffed-up nostrils, headache and pain back of the eyes, take sufficient amount of the leaves of the tree and have them pounded thoroughly. The mixture is then taken and put in a container with sufficient amount of water added to it. Put in four red-hot stones and, as the liquid steams, the patient sits before the container inhaling the steam. Cover the patient with tapa as for steam bath, shutting up all openings that may allow the steam to escape. The patient then opens his mouth and takes the fumes in. As the liquid cools down, the entire body, from head to foot, is bathed with it. This treatment is taken morning and evening and for five successive times. Spring water should be the regular drink.

For chills and sever pain at the joints, take a big quantity of the "ahi-ahi" leaves with two handfuls of the roots and a hatful of wild "maile" and the large-leaf "maile" ("mailue kaluhea"). Pound these thoroughly and add sufficient amount of water to the mixture. Then put in four red-hot stones, stirring the entire mixture slowly while the steam increases in volume. Cover the patient with "tapa" and allow the steam to get all over the entire body as before. As the water cools down, bathe the entire body, from head to foot, with it. This done, the patient lies on his back with sufficient cover over him and goes to sleep. This is done in the morning. At about noon, when the sun is hot, he goes and bathes himself in salt water. This is followed with a sun bath on hot sand. This is repeated five times and at equal intervals. Then he returns to his home and takes hot roast potato (cooked over the charcoal) broiled fish and "luau" (cooked taro leaf) for his lunch. Proper laxative should be taken for internal cleansing.

11. AHI-HI (LAU-AWA). (No specimen for identification.)

This tree grows and appears the same as the "Ah-hi-ku-makua." The leaves, however, are smaller than those of the "ahi-hi-ku-makua." The leaves, again, are somewhat twisted and when crushed throws out powerful and fragrant odor. The plant is very hard to get owing to its scarcity. But it may be found among the Hilo mountains and at Halemano on Oahu; also at Waimea, Palolo, Oahu; Kilohana overlooking Hanalei, and at Namolokama, Kauai; and among the hills of Hana, Kipahulu to Keanae, Maui.

As a medicine its value is like that of the "ahihi-ku-makua" and so is its preparation and application. But, in addition, its bud is useful for children about the age of five or six years who are afflicted with general debility, usually arising from bad stomach and from constipation. In preparing it take eight buds and have them chewed with cocoanut. Swallow the juice only, throwing the solid matter away. This is done twice a day for five days in succession. After that time, take the *Ipomea dissecta* for a laxative—the root chewed with white sugar cane.

12. AHINAHINA. (*Artemisis Australis* var. *Escholsiana*)

This herb grows in abundance on nearly all the mountains of the Hawaiian Islands. It is found at Makana, Kauai; Kalihi, Manoa, Waialua, Oahu. Its leaves are fragrant like those of the fruit-bearing "koa" and are often woven into wreaths.

This remedy is good for high fever (dry fever, having no perspiration), with dizziness afflicting the head; it is also good for asthma or lung trouble.

For high fever take two hatfuls (men's hat) quantity of the leaves of the herb, also its trunk and roots, and pound them thoroughly. Add to this mixture the bark of four roots of the *Ipomea pes-caprae*, with two handfuls of the "naio" (dried) ashes. Add sufficient amount of water, and heat the whole with eight hot stones. As the steam arises, put the patient at the side of the container holding the boiling liquid and give him a steam bath. When the medicine water cools down to the right temperature, bathe the patient with it. This treatment is given five successive times, after which the laxative, *Ipomea dissecta*, is taken to clean the bowels. Fresh poi, broiled fish, "luau" and "kukui"-nut may be taken as food while the patient, for five successive days remains in quietness and in a restful attitude.

For lung trouble and hard breathing take two hatfuls (men's size) of the "hinahina" leaves with two half-ripe *Morinda citrifolia* fruits together with a handful of the stems of the *peperomia* spp. and three segments of white sugar cane. These are pounded together with sufficient amount of spring water. Then the mixture is put into the *Cyperus laevigata* fibers, carefully and finely done without the use of water; and through these fibers the liquid of the mixture is pressed out and cleaned. This liquid is then mixed with "huamoa" potato or the "mohihi" potato, while it is steaming. This is eaten for three successive days. After that, the luau (cooked taro leaves), the "kuikui"-nut and broiled fish are eaten to close the treatment. The *Campylotheca* tea is taken internally for drinking water for eight successive days. As usual, the *Ipomea dissecta* laxative is taken for internal cleaning.

13. HINAHINA KU-KAHAKAI. (No specimen for identification.)

This is a creeping plant and grows abundantly along the shore. It resembles the "hinahina-ku-pali" in many ways. It has white flowers. Unlike those of the "hinahina-ku-pali," the flowers and leaves are not fragrant.

This remedy is used for the cure of general debility, lung trouble, and the diseases of the sexual and other vital organs.

In preparing it, take sufficient quantity (a hatful) of its flowers and leaves; an equal amount of "popolo" berries; one piece of the "ohia" bark the size of the palm of the hand; one "kukui"-nut roasted thoroughly; three segments of the white sugar cane; and two medium-size clusters of "kukui" flowers. Pound these thoroughly together until mixed and then press the juice out with the fine fibers of the *Cyperus laevigata*. The cleaned liquid, in sufficient amount (a glassful) is then taken internally three times a day. The *Campylotheca* tea is taken in place of water.

For asthma and kindred troubles, and for womb or vaginal complications, take ten plants,—root, leaves, and all—eight pieces of the tap root bark of the "hialoa" plant, four half-ripe fruits of the *Morinda citrifolia*, four segments of the white sugar cane, a hatful of the leaves, fruit and flowers of the "naio." Pound these until thoroughly mixed and then press the juice out with the finely prepared fibers of the *Cyperus laevigata*. Put in one red hot stone, stirring the liquid slowly until cooked, and using four "lau-i" buds in the liquid while it is being stirred. As the liquid cools, remove the stone. The patient then lies down facing a hard floor with a cushion under the chest (should the trouble be in the lungs or under the *mons veneris* if the affliction is around the sexual organ of the female.)

The liquid is then taken internally. This is done morning and evening for five successive times. Between the treatments the green "popolo" leaves are eaten. Brackish or light salty water should be taken as drink. Meat is prohibited. Broiled fish or that cooked in "ti"-leaf, "luau," potato leaves cooked either by roasting or boiling, "popolo" leaves, somewhat sour poi, potato and breadfruit are suitable articles of food for the patient.

14. AHINA-KUAHIWI or KA-APE-APE. (No specimen for identification.)

This herb is found on Haleakala, at Keanae and Nahiki Mountains, Maui; at Konahuanui, Kuahiwiwo, Manoa, Kaliuwaa, Kukaniloko and Waimea mountains, Oahu; at Wainiha, Hanalei, Lihue and at Kilohana on the side facing Hanalei, Kauai; and, in some parts of Hawaii. This remedy is usully applied to cases of general debility and of stomach trouble. The whole plant is used for medicine. In preparing it, take the entire plant and dry it thoroughly and then burn it to ashes. Take the fully matured "opihi" shell for the measure (this is the size of a tablespoon) and take four shells full of the ashes of the plant and pour it into the cleaned liquid from a mixture of four hatfuls of *Peperomia* spp. stems thoroughly pounded together with two pieces of mountain apple bark, one *Morina citrifolia* fruit that is fully matured and almost ripening, to segments of white sugar cane, and the bark of four "popolo" roots.

Take one shell-ful of the liquid internally three times a day. This remedy is good for children from one month to six years old. When applied to adults, the juice from the taproot bark of the *Waltheria americana* should be added. When applying to children, the milk from the meat of fully matured cocoanut should be given to them after the remedy is taken. The ripe leaves of the "ahina" is helpful in drawing inflammation from rheumatic knee and joints of the legs. The leaves are taken and laid over the afflicted parts and allowed to remain there for some time.

15. AKALA or AKALAKALA. (*Rubus hawaiiansis* and *R. macraei*.)

This is a creeping plant, the vine spreading here and there as it grows. It is found chiefly among the highlands, hills and mountains. In appearance, it resembles the "ohelo" and its leaves are like those of the "maile."

Its use as a remedy is confined chiefly to such troubles as scaly scalp, burning within the bosom and vomiting.

For scaly scalp take the entire plant and dry it thoroughly. At the same time a whole tobacco leaf is thoroughly dried. Both of these are separately burned to ashes. In the meantime, a container, holding about a quart of water, is being placed out in the hot sun to warm the water. When ready for use, the ashes of this herb, together with the tobacco ashes, are thrown into the warm water and stirred until thoroughly mixed. The head is then washed with the mixture, rubbing it into the scalp. One or two treatments are sufficient to rid the head of this affliction.

For the burning effect in the chest take about a tablespoonful (one "opihi" shell) of the ashes of the "akala" and pour it into an equal amount of papaia meat—the portion taken from the base of the fruit. This mixture is eaten, followed by sufficient amount of water. Two treatments are sufficient to bring about absolute cure with no repetition of the trouble following.

For vomiting, take a similar amount of the ashes of the plant and put it into an equal amount of either poi or potato. The mixture is then eaten, followed by chewing two small lumps of Hawaiian salt and drinking about a glass of water ("apu," as mentioned here, holds about a glass or more of water).

16. AKIA LAUNUI or AKIA PENU or AKIA MANALO or AKEA.
(*Winstroemia* sspp.)

This herb grows most abundantly on Molokai. It also grows among some of the mountains on Hawaii and Maui and at Mokuleia, Waialua and other places on Oahu. It may be found on Kauai.

It is a low-growing plant having large, thick leaves. It contains considerable slimy sap water and, for this reason, it is frequently used for laxative.

In preparing it take four plants, one-half dried cocoanut, one-half segment of the white sugar cane and have these pounded together thoroughly. The juice of this mixture is then squeezed out and cleansed. Take about a tablespoonful of the liquid thus formed and pour it into an opening made in the center of a charcoal-roasted sweet potato. This filled, the liquid is covered and allowed to soak into the potato. The potato is then eaten and the mixture will act as a laxative for the bowels. Should its action be more than is needed, then take four lumps of the Hawaiian starch and chew them. This is followed by drinking about a glass full of water. Take liberal quantity of the *Campylotheca* spp. tea.

For a stubborn case of asthma take four plants, a hatful of the "naio" leaves and buds, two pieces of mountain apple bark, the bark of four roots of the *Waltheria americana*, half of partly dried cocoanut meat, one and a half segments (medium size) of white sugar cane. Pound these together thoroughly and squeeze the juice into a container and clean it with the finely prepared fibers of the *Cyperus laevigata*. Take the liquid cold with face down on hard floor and a cushion under the abdomen. Take this treatment morning and evening for five successive times. Fish having dark flesh, such as the "aku," "kawakawa," "akule," "opelu," etc., should not be eaten; nor the "luau," or taro leaf. Poi not more than a day and a half or two days old is good, also vegetables cooked with heated stones.

17. AHUAWA. (*Cyperus laevigata.*)

This plant grows wildly in swamps like those at Waikiki and elsewhere throughout the Hawaiian Islands. The flowers with their long stems are valuable. It grows in large bunches. Its leaves are slender and long, having cutting edge on both sides. The fiber of the stem is frequently woven into strings and ropes for various purposes and is largely used for liquid cleaning purposes,—the fiber being finely combed and folded to such thickness as would collect and remove all impurities in the liquid passing thru it.

The long stem or stalk with the flowers of the "ahuawa" are employed for the cure of general debility. Take two stalks with their flowers and dry them thoroughly. Then burn them to ashes—have enough, if necessary, to fill about a tablespoon. Take four young kukui nuts and accumulate in a container, the juice that issues from where the nuts are broken off from their stems. The ashes and the "kukui" juice are then mixed and rubbed on the tongue morning and evening.

There are two kinds of physical debility; one is of a temporary nature and the other continuous, producing a thick white coating on the tongue almost all the time. In case the two mingle, then add to the above mixture a thoroughly roasted "kukui"-nut (*Aleurites moluccana*) powdered and applied in the same manner.

This remedy is also good for burning affliction within the penis or certain burning disease of the male-organ. The stalk is partly dried and crushed to fine particles. This is put into about a handful of reddish Hawaiian clay, dried and powdered. To this add about a quart of spring water. Then take a mouthful of chewed "awa"-root (*Piper methysticum*) and mix it in about a quart of spring water. The two are mixed together and taken internally. This is followed by chewing a segment of white sugar-cane. The remedy is taken morning and evening for five successive times, or days. Between times, considerable spring water should be taken— about four or five glasses each time and at least five or more times a day.

Deep cuts, bad boils, ulcers of the skin, and other skin diseases can be cured with the use of the "ahu-awa" powder, especially when the "lama-kuahiwi" (no scientific name given) powder is added to it, thus increasing its absorbing and drying power in the process of healing. By gradually snuffing into the nostrils the "ahu-awa" powder, a hard cold in the head can be destroyed.

18. AKAAKAI. (Onion, common variety.)

The onion is used in the different mixtures of remedies for the cure of such diseases as tuberculosis, colds and venereal diseases. It is in the mixtures given below that the different uses of the onion is mentioned.

19. AKAAKAI (KIKANIA). (Onion, common variety.)

This variety is smaller than the former and is used for ear trouble. Take one bulb, a bit of "olena" (*Curcuma louza*) and four very young shoots of the "ti"-plant ("la'i"), using the white portion only. All these are pounded together and put into the hollow of finely drawn cocoanut fibers. The patient then lies on his side with the afflicted ear up. The fiber container is put over the ear and the liquid from the mixture is then pressed out, allowing two or three drops to fall into the ear, at the same time pressing around the base with the thumb and forefinger in order to aid the remedy in getting to the troubled part. The application is made two or three times a day and for five days in succession. Where the cure is realized before the fifth day, further application is not necessary.

20. AKAAKAI-MAHINA. (No specimen for identification.)

The variety grows in swamps and on plains. It is low, having thick leaves and large fruit resembling the appearance of thumb and forefinger in open position. The interior portion of the plant is useful for sore-throat.

In preparing the remedy, take four bulbs and leave them in a damp place. As they grow, take the young shoots and allow them to wither. Then pound them with twenty fully matured "popolo" leaves and the bark of four roots of the *Waltheria americana* and two pickings of Hawaiian salt. The mixture is then put into the finely prepared fibers of the *Cyperus laevigata* and the liquid from it is pressed out and cleaned. This liquid in sufficient amount is then taken into the mouth for a gargle. The whole is used each time, a new mixture being provided at each application. Gargle morning and evening for five days in succession. This done, a sufficient amount of salt water from the ocean is warmed and taken in for a thorough washing out of the bowels. For diet during the treatment, take somewhat fermented poi or sour potato and breadfruit with broiled fish. Drink *Campylotheca* spp. tea for drinking water.

21. AKAAKAI NAKU or NEKI. (No scientific name given.)

This reed grows most abundantly in swamps and along streams and in taro patches. The dried reeds are woven into hats and mats. The root of the reed is the portion used for medicine.

For gripping pain of the stomach or intestines and for internal hemorrhage, take four handfuls of its roots, the meat of one green "kukui" nut, eight "kukui" nut flowers, one half-ripe *Morinda citrifolia* fruit, and one segment of white sugar-cane. Thoroughly pound these together and squeeze out the liquid from this mixture. Clean it thoroughly and allow it to stand in a container for awhile. Then drop into it a red-hot stone. As the foam begins to gather, drink it down slowly. This is done morning and evening and for five times in succession. Take *Campylotheca* spp. tea for drink; fresh poi and broiled fish for food; warmed salt water from the ocean for laxative.

22. AKI-AKI or MANIENIE-MAHIKIHIKI.

(*Stenotaphrum americanum*) (Buffalo grass)

This is a thick, stubby grass that creeps as it grows. It abounds in places near the beach and on plains.

This remedy is most effective in case of excessive catamenia. Take a hatful of the "akiaki" leaves, including stem, and an equal amount of *Peperomia* spp. stems. In the meantime, soak in about two pints of water (spring water), a lump of good red Hawaiian clay. Pound the "akiaki" and the "alaalawainui" together thoroughly and then, through the finely drawn cocoanut fibers, squeeze out the juice of this mixture and empty it into the clay solution. Mix the whole thoroughly and add the white of an egg. After stirring the whole thing thoroughly, the patient drinks it down. This is followed by the eating of a medium-sized charcoal, roasted sweet potato, and four bits of Hawaiian salt. The treatment is taken morning and evening for five successive times. No meat should be eaten. Charcoal cooked fish is good during the treatment.

When the remedy takes effect, the symptoms are these: the eyes become heavy and the patient becomes somewhat dizzy and sleepy. Sneezing becomes frequent.

After the treatment, sufficient quantity of ocean salt water should be taken to clean out the bowels.

The ashes of the "akiaki" leaves are beneficial for sores on babies; also for navel sores. When mixed with the secretion of two young "kukui" nuts, it becomes effective for ulcers on the skin and for excessive saliva from babies' mouths. For an afterbirth treatment, the ashes of this grass is very healing to the vagina and neighboring parts.

23. A-KOKO or AKO-KOKO. (*Euphorbia multiformis.*)

This is a low-growing and somewhat dwarfed-looking plant, having whitish trunk with thick leaves. For general debility of the body the bud, as well as the leaf, is beneficial.

For a month-old baby take two buds and have the mother chew them and give the mixture to the baby. For a baby three months old give four buds, and so on till the age of six months.

Again: It is a regular practice for the mother to chew eight buds or leaves of the "akoko" and have the babe take it through her milk. When it is six months old, the mother takes about sixteen buds or leaves. She continues this until the offspring leaves the breast. In taking the leaves or buds, however, a piece of roasted cocoanut should be eaten together. The remedy is a good laxative for the mother. It also stimulates considerable appetite, which is most helpful in milk production. For a laxative, it should be taken with roasted sweet potato.

For dry breast, take about a tablespoonful of the "akoko" milk and pour it on a mixture of thoroughly cooked young taro leaves (eight in number for medium-size ones, and four and a half for full-size ones), and a thoroughly cooked "kukui" nut (half size), mashed together on a board. After mixing, the mother takes the whole thing internally either with poi or sweet potato and this is followed by a drink of water. This remedy is taken for five successive days. Other articles of food may be taken, but only after the "luau" part of the medicine is taken. For scrofulous lumps, take a tablespoonful of the "akoko" milk and mix this with an equal amount of powdered *Cyperus laevigata* (root and stalk). The mixture is then applied to the sore by covering it. Then the patient sits where the rays of the sun could squarely strike the sore and allow the medicine to dry on it. This is done morning and evening.

For female weaknesses about the reproductive organ, and, for building up the body, the "akoko" may be depended upon to do the work. For female weaknesses, take a hatful of the buds and leaves; an equal amount of "lehua" buds; two good-sized pieces of the mountain apple bark; four half-ripe *Morinda citrifolia* fruits; three segments of white sugar-cane; a hatful of the *Peperomia* stems. Pound these together thoroughly and press the juice out into a container and have it cleaned in the usual method. In the meantime thoroughly mix about a tablespoonful of Hawaiian starch. Two red-hot stones are then placed in the "akoko" mixture and, as it steams, the starch is gradually poured into it and the whole thing is stirred. After the liquid cools down to the right temperature, the patient lies down on the hard floor, face down, with a cushion supporting the abdomen. The liquid is then taken internally, followed by the chewing of a piece of dried cocoanut meat. The eating of meat is prohibited during the treatment; only the white-fleshed fish can be eaten.

24. AKO-LEA or PAKIKAWAIO or KA'EKOLEA or ALAALAI.
(*Phegopteris.*)

This herb grows extensively among the mountains of the Hawaiian islands. The leaves are large, having the shape of the palm of the hand. Its roots, like those of the tree-fern, are frequently cooked for food. The young shoot or bud and the trunk of this herb are employed for the purpose of restoring lost appetite. In preparing it, take that part of the trunk that is stubby, having numerous segments, and scrape off the bark with "opihi" shell until the central portion is exposed. This, again, is scraped until an amount equal to that of a medium-sized bowl is obtained. Have eight young taro leaves cooked in the meantime, also one "kukui" nut, the latter being pounded to that fineness that would mix. These three, the "akolea" pulp, the cooked taro leaves and the "kukui," are then thrown together and thoroughly stirred. The mixture is then eaten with a day-old poi or mashed sweet potato. This is repeated until the appetite for poi and fish is restored.

After five days the "koali" (*Ipomea dissecta*) is taken as a laxative for internal cleaning. In preparing it, take two vines at arm's length and as large around the vine as the forefinger, and pound these thoroughly with a segment of the white sugar-cane. The juice from this mixture is then squeezed out and cleansed and this is mixed with the white of an egg. The patient then drinks the mixture down, if possible, in its raw state. If not, a red-hot stone is dropped into the liquid and, after it is cooked and cooled to the right temperature, it is taken down. Should the bowels move too freely a lump of Hawaiian starch must be secured and dissolved in sufficient amount of water. This is taken as a drink, which readily relieves the patient.

During childbirth, this remedy is most helpful. The inside of the trunk is scraped until a sufficient quantity (about a large glassful) is secured. In the meantime four young taro leaves are cooked and made ready on a board. The two are then mixed with about a glassful of spring water, and given to the patient. Or take four buds of the "ako-lea" and cook it with the young taro leaves. These are mixed and then eaten. At the same time, the patient takes the prepared "akolea" (the scraping mixed with spring water) and eats that, too,—the same way that soup is taken.

25. A-LAA. (*Sideroxylon*)

This tree grows in the mountains of all the islands, except, perhaps, the mountains of the Island of Hawaii. Its leaves are large like those of the *Hibiscus tiliaceus*. Its trunk is like that of the "lama." Its bark, leaves and wood, in dry state, are usually mixed with other herbs for producing strong remedies.

For general debility and strong fever, the following mixture is used: Two hatsful of leaves; an equal amount of bark, the pieces being the size of the palm of the hand; one "olena" (*Curcuma louza*) bulb or root; four pickings of Hawaiian salt. Pound these together thoroughly and add eight cups of water and stir the whole until mixed. This is strained and cleaned and then applied to the entire body from head to foot, rubbing in as the application is made. The application is made three times a day, taking internally about a tablespoonful of the liquid every now and then. Use spring water for drinking and *Ipomea dissecta* for a laxative.

26. ALA-ALA-PU-LOA. (*Waltheria americana*)

This is a low-growing plant. Its leaves are thick and succulent, very breakable and having the shape of the mountain apple leaves. It grows in damp ground. It is commonly found at Kukaniloko, Kuai-kua, Nuuanu, Manoa and Kaliuwaa, Oahu. It is also found at Hamakua, Keanae, Maui; also in some parts of Hawaii and Kauai. In taste, it is puckery, and it is largely employed in the cure of asthma.

In preparing it, take one hatful of the buds and leaves of the "alaala-puloa"; eight roots; half a hatful of "akoko" buds, and two segments of red sugar-cane. Pound these thoroughly and then add about two pints of water. Mix the whole thing carefully and then strain it. Then add to the cleaned liquid about two tablespoonfuls of burnt "ti"-root juice. The entire content is then poured into a narrow-neck gourd container and thoroughly shaken. This done, the patient then drinks about a tablespoonful of the liquid. This is done three times a day. At the end, "koali" laxative is taken for internal cleaning.

27. ALA-ALA-WAIONUI-PEHU. (*Peperomia* spp.)

This herb grows thickly and at about an arm's length in height. Its leaves are round and thick and its trunk is similar to that of the castor-oil plant, having very fine hairs and of reddish color. The wood is somewnat brittle and, therefore, very easy to break. This herb is very helpful to a newly born baby. For one who is five days old, the mother may take two buds and chew them with eight "ilima" (*Sida* spp.) flowers. The mixture is then given to the baby. The slimy or slippery character of the mixture acts as a soft and easy laxative for the child's bowels, and it removes from them the darkened waste which, for days, has accumulated. This internal cleaning paves the way for the child to take the mother's milk and does away with a condition which might be very disturbing to the constitution. This treatment should be given morning and evening.

For general debility, take a handful of the stems stripped of their leaves; two pieces (each piece being the size of the palm of the hand) of mountain apple bark; four segments of the white sugar-cane; two branches of "kukui" flowers; one burnt "kukui"-nut and two onions. Pound these together thoroughly and then add to the mixture the powdered substance of crushed fresh *Cyperus laevigata* stalks. The mixture is then strained and made ready for use.

For a baby forty days old, a half-spoonful is sufficient for drinking at one time. For one older than this, a whole tablespoonful may be taken. The same amount may be given to one five months old. In all cases, the remedy must be well shaken before drinking it. Never allow a single mixture to stand for more than three days. Should it be found necessary to keep it on hand for a longer period of time, then two tablespoonfuls of burnt "ti"-root juice should be mixed with it. The treatment is applied three times a day and as long as necessary. At the end, a laxative must be taken.

For wasting away of the body and for general weakness, take a hatful of the stems of the herb; one young shoot of the tree fern; eight shoots of *Pandanus odoratissimus* roots; two pieces (the size of the palm of the hand) of mountain apple bark; three segments of white sugar-cane; two fully matured *Morinda citrifolia* fruits. Pound these together thoroughly and then have the juice of the mixture strained and cleaned. Put into the liquid thus prepared one red-hot stone. Stir it as it cooks and then allow it to cool. At the right temperature, the patient drinks the whole of it, after which he eats two "iholena" bananas and then takes a drink of water. This remedy is taken morning and evening for five consecutive days. White flesh fish, broiled on charcoal, and "kukui"-nut, together with young taro leaf that is thoroughly cooked, should be taken for food. Boiled pure salt water from the ocean should be taken as a laxative after the treatment.

For pulmonary diseases, take a hatful of the herbs; four tubers of the "four o'clock," or twilight flower plant; two pieces of the *Morinda citrifolia* bark the size of the palm of the hand; two young *Cibatium vhamissoi* Kaulf. shoots; four segments of the white sugar-cane, and four branches of "kukui" flowers. Pound these thoroughly and then mix with about a quart of water. Strain this mixture and then take it internally, morning and evening, for five consecutive days. At the end, take the "kowali" (*Ipomea dissecta*) for laxative.

For affliction about the generative or sexual organ of the female, take the entire plant—roots, leaves, trunks, flowers and all—about a quartful of the *Euphorbia multiformis* buds; a half of matured and fresh cocoanut; four stems and shoots of the "kikawaioa." Pound these thoroughly together and then pour into the mixture half of a cocoanut (approaching maturity) milk. Strain the entire contents. The patient then drinks down the cleaned liquid from the mixture. In the meantime, the scraping from a half-ripe "lele" banana is being cooked in "ti"-leaf, and this is eaten immediately after the "alaalawainui" (*Peperomia* spp.) medicine is taken. The treatment is taken morning and evening for five consecutive days, and it must be begun eight days before the monthly menstruation takes place.

28. ALA-ALA-WAI-NUI POHINA (female). (No specimen for identification.)

This is a low-growing plant, having gray leaves similar to those of the "alaalawainui pehu" (*Peperomia* spp.) and flowers of grayish-white color. It grows at Waimea and Mana, Kauai; also at Puako, Kawaihae, Puna, and Kau, Hawaii. It grows at the lee of Maui; at Molokai and Lanai; at Waimanalo, Kaena and Waialua, on Oahu.

This remedy is largely employed for the cure of children's general debility; also for the cure of scrofulous swellings and ulcers.

For a baby affected with general debility, say after ten days old, the mother takes four flowers, using just the very core, chews them and feeds the baby with the mixture. This is done once a day for five consecutive days, usually before feeding. For a baby of six months or a year old, feed with a mixture of eight flowers (using only the core), followed by the eating of roasted potato and the mother's milk. Should the bowels move too freely, the child should be given four medium-sized lumps of Hawaiian starch to dissolve in its mouth. Poi may be given as well as the mother's milk. The mother must take laxative in order to insure a healthy system. Four green leaves, or the dry ones, of the "akoko" (*Euphorbia multiformis*) together with a piece of dry cocoanut make a very satisfactory medicine for cleaning the bowels.

For bad cases of asthma, take a hatful of the plant and an equal amount of the "alaalawainui pehu" (*Peperomia* spp.) ; two pieces of the mountain apple bark; one partly dried cocoanut; two matured fruits of the *Morinda citrifolia*, and two segments of white sugar-cane. Pound these thoroughly together and then strain the liquid from this mixture and give it to the patient to drink. This is followed by the eating of half of four "iholena" bananas. This treatment should be taken before breakfast and supper for five consecutive days. Partly fermented poi with white flesh fish broiled over charcoal together with cooked young taro leaves, "kukui"-nut, young potato leaves should be eaten as food, with spring water for drink.

For irregular monthly periods of women and for swollen womb, the "alaalawainui pohina" (*Peperomia*) is very effective. Take three hatfuls of the leaves and stems of the plant; eight buds and two leaves (below the bud) of the "akoko" (*Euphorbia multiformis*); eight "kanawao" (*Cyrtandra* sp, white variety) fruits; four young shoots of the "amau" (tree fern, or *Sadleria cyathecides*) and a segment of red sugar-cane. Pound these thoroughly and strain the juice therefrom into a container and have it cleaned. Then scrape into it the bark and wood of the "kikawaioa" at the same time crushing the soft bud of the plant in the mixture. The patient then lies down with the chest supported by blankets. He takes the mixture and drinks it. At the same time he eats, little by little, the "piaaaoa" banana until four are taken. Spring water should be taken for drink and six "pilikai" (*Argyreia tiliaefolia*) seeds crushed to powder, for laxative.

29. ALAEA or KUMAUNA. (*Splenium horridum*)

This tree grows like the "noni" (*Morinda citrifolia*). Its fruit is like the "kamani" fruit. In this fruit is a red slimy juice which is employed in dyeing the "kapa." The color is waterproof.

The dry wood of this tree is used for those subjected to fainting spells accompanied by stiffened muscles.

Scrape the wood until a tablespoonful is obtained and then pour it into about two pints of water. Take eight blades of the buffalo grass (*Stenotaphrum americanum*) and crush them between the thumb and forefinger, with four lumps of Hawaiian salt. Then have the patient take this entire mixture internally at the same time rubbing some on the afflicted part of the body.

For sore mouth, take four buds and chew them with the burnt peel (the black or scorched part being scraped off) of a potato. This is followed by a drink of water.

For impure blood, take two pieces of the "alaea" (*Asplenium horridum*) bark; two of the mountain apple; two of the breadfruit; one hatful of the "kookoolau" (*Campylotheca* spp.) leaves and flowers only; four pieces of the "uhaloa" (*Waltheria americana*) bark; four tap-root bark of the "aukoi" (*Cassia occidentalis*); four segments of the white sugar-cane.

Pound these together thoroughly with about a quart of cocoanut milk. The juice or liquid coming from this mixture is then strained into a container into which two red-hot stones are put to cook the liquid. Should it be necessary to prolong the use of a single mixture to avoid repetition of the trouble of fixing it, then add the strong juice of the "ti"-root. A tablespoonful of this liquid is taken three times a day until the mixture is consumed. The patient should not eat raw fish or fish having dark flesh. Charcoal broiled fish, fish cooked with "ti"-leaves, together with "kukui"-nut, young taro leaves, young potato leaves and poi just beginning to ferment are good articles of food. Potato is also a good food. The "kookoolau" (*Campylotheca*) tea should be taken as drink regularly.

30. ALAEA (red clay)   (No specimen.)

This clay is red in color and is very effective in cases of excessive menstruation, diseased womb, difficulties in monthly periods of women, strong asthma, and general debility and kindred troubles. In applying, the clay is not taken alone but is mixed with other things of medicinal value.

For the general debility of the body as well as for the lung and kindred troubles of the chest, take a lump of clay the size of a pear fruit and let it stand in a half-quart of water. Take a hatful of the *Peperomia* spp. stems; an equal amount of the "lehua" buds; a handful of "kohekohe" (small reeds growing in bunches in taro patches); a piece of the mountain apple bark; two branches of the "kukui" flowers and two segments of the white sugarcane. Pound these together thoroughly and then mix the whole with the soaked clay. Then strain the entire content until the liquid from it is clean. This is then taken internally in its raw state. This is done morning and evening for five consecutive days, eating a piece of cocoanut after each dose is taken.

Poi and charcoal broiled fish are good articles of food for this treatment. Should the patient want raw fish, "oio" and "ala" can be taken. Young taro leaves with "kukui"-nut and potato and "popolo" leaves are good for vegetables.

For laxative take six "pilikai" seeds. These are crushed and then powdered to the condition suitable for taking internally. In some instances, the clay is taken by itself and eaten. This is followed by a drink of water.

This clay is frequently used in coloring eating salt, and in this way the commonly known red salt is made.

31. ALANI-KUAHIWI.   (*Pelea* spp.)

This herb grows among the mountains of Konahuanui, Kaliuwaa, Waoala, Manoa and Palolo, Oahu; of Lahainaluna, Iao, Haleakala, Keanae and Nahiku, Maui; of Waipio, at Piihonua, Hilo; of Waimanu, Hawaii; of Kawaikini, Alakai, Maia o Laau and Maunahina, Kauai. The leaves of this plant are similar to those of the regular orange and so is the trunk and the entire tree. Its flowers are somewhat yellowish. The leaves and flowers are fragrant but the bark is very bitter.

The "alani" is the Hawaiian beauty remedy and is dedicated to the exclusive use of the Kings and Queens and their sons and daughters. The leaves, in sufficient quantity, are taken and laid on the bed, covering the space, say, from the neck to the feet. A sheeting of "tapa," tightly drawn, is laid over the leaves. In the meantime, twenty leaves are allowed to remain in the water overnight and placed in the sun during the day. This is for bathing. Towards evening, the royal child, or the one chosen for beauty, is given a bath of this water. In it is put the "alani" flowers. After the bath the child is fed on fattening ration. After feeding, and when the child becomes sleepy, it is placed in the bed covered with the "alani" leaves. This is repeated for five consecutive days. The bedding is then changed, the old "alani" leaves are removed and new ones take their place, and the process continues from that point on for five days more. Not only does this treatment improve the appearance, but it makes the skin immune to certain diseases, especially skin diseases.

The young shoot or bud is usually cut and the top portion thrown away, while the lower portion is kept. This is a good remedy for children having general debility. For babies ten days old, two of the lower halves of the buds are given; for those three months old, four; and from that time on they are given quantities proportionate to their age.

For purifying the blood, take four pieces of the "alani" bark the size of the palm of the hand; an equal amount of the "koa" (the kind out of which the canoe is made) bark; a hatful of the "lehua" buds; mountain apple bark having the same quantity as that if the "alani" bark; six *Waltheria americana* tap-root bark and four segments of the red sugar-cane.

Pound these thoroughly together and put the mixture into a container. Pour into the container about a quartful of water and mix the whole thoroughly. Then put into the mixture about four red-hot stones and cover the entire contents tightly so that the steam may remain within the container. When the content is thoroughly cooked add to it about two tablespoonsful of the "ti"-juice. This is very bitter. Then strain the liquid thoroughly and put it into a container or bottle. Take a mouthful of this liquid at a time, either before or after meals, and take it three times a day. Fish, broiled over the charcoal or cooked in "ti"-leaves, or cooked with heated stones, including "luau," or cooked young taro leaves, cooked young potato leaves, potato, taro and banana, are good articles of food to take during the treatment. At the end, take forty matured *Morinda citrifolia* fruits and use their juice for injection to clean the bowels.

32. A-MAU-MAU or A-MAU.   (*Sadleria cyatheoedes*)

This plant is found among the mountains of the Hawaiian Islands. Its use as a medicine is for the purpose of curing asthma and kindred troubles.

Take the trunk and scrape off the outside until the soft interior is exposed. Then lay this portion out in the hot sun, most preferably on stones where the sun strikes hard. When it gets brown and thoroughly dried and somewhat brittle, grind it into powder on a hard board. In the meantime, take eight tap-root barks of the *Waltheria americana*, eight "popolo" roots; one bark of the "kuikui"; one sweet potato about the size of the palm of the hand; two segments of white sugar-cane. These are thoroughly pounded together and the juice strained and cleaned. The powdered "amau" and the juice thus obtained are put together in a container and a red hot stone is put into the mixture to cook it. After it is cooled it is taken morning and evening for five consecutive times.

For the drinking water, it is well to put into it the "amau" dust. But the water should be boiled and enough should be prepared to last a day's treatment. It should be taken when the water is warm. It may be mentioned here that the young shoot of the "amau" is good for lung troubles.

This should be mixed as follows: Four "amau" shoots; a hatful of the *Peperomia* spp. stems; an equal amount of the *Peperomia* spp. flowers; about two pints filled with "lehua" buds; two fully matured *Morinda citrifolia* fruits and two segments of the white sugar-cane. Pound these thoroughly together and strain the juice into a container. This comprises one dose. This is taken in the morning. In the evening another is taken and this is repeated for five consecutive times. Maintain regular exercise morning and evening.

For bringing boils, blind pimples and similar afflictions to a head and for bringing the puss outside, the "amau" is very helpful. Take one piece of "amau"; a piece of "kukui" bark; half of the "kukui" nut meat; and four lumps of Hawaiian salt. Pound these thoroughly together and gather the entire mixture into a sieve or cocoanut fiber strainer. As the juice from it is squeezed out, it is rubbed over the boil, leaving a circular space where the head appears. The patient then sits out where the boil can readily be exposed to the sun. As the remedy dries up it contracts, thus bringing pressure around the boil and forcing the puss to move toward the uncovered spot. The head of the boil then appears and enlarges until it bursts open. Together with this use of the "amau," poi and "nona" are frequently employed.

As a drink "amau" powder is frequently used. About a tablespoonful of it is put in about a quart of boiling water and is prepared like coffee or tea.

33. APE KEOKEO or APII.   (*Alocasia macrorrhiza*)

This plant, which resembles the taro, is found everywhere and is frequently planted as a decorative plant. Its chief uses are: the healing of severe burns; love-making by "kahunas" and curing stomach-ache.

For a severe burn take a piece of the "ape"-taro about the size of the forefinger. Pound this thoroughly. In the meantime, half of a dried cocoanut and two stalks of the *Cyperus laevigata* are being burnt to ashes. Combine these three things and mix them in the white of one egg. This done, the mixture is then spread over the burn.

For love-making, the "kahunas" have used this white "ape" for a sort of a stimulant, thus effecting a constant reminder to the one desired of the presence or wish of his or her admirer.

For acute pain in the stomach or bowels, take a piece of the "ape" the size of the forefinger; a quart full of the leaves and flowers of the "kookoolau" (*Campylotheca*) plant and pound together thoroughly. Add to this mixture about a quart of water and, after stirring the whole content together, strain it and take internally. This will act as a laxative and an appetizer. Refrain from eating salty foods. Use as much of the remedy as possible. To make the remedy more effective, cooked young taro leaves and the slimy "kikawaioa" may be added while mixing.

34. APE-HIWA or APE-ELEELE.   (No specimen.)

This, in all details, resembles the "ape-keokeo" except it is dark in color. This plant has very little medicinal value. So far as is known, its use is confined to the destruction of worms which cause considerable annoyance to the rectum. In preparing it take a piece of the "ape-hiwa"; four *Waltheria americana* leaves; the meat of one "kukui"-nut and pound together thoroughly. The juice is then squeezed out and strained and then applied by forcing it to the afflicted part of the rectum. Do this morning and evening.

35. AWA.   (*Piper methysticum*)

There are many different kinds of "awa." They are known by their leaves, bark and roots. Its use as a medicine is confined chiefly to the cure of sleeplessness and general debility of the body. In preparing it, take the "awa" and dry it in the sun. When it is partly dried, wash it clean and chop it to pieces of convenient size. These pieces are either chewed or pounded. If chewed, then allow five mouthfuls of the thoroughly chewed "awa" for a dose. This is taken and mixed in about a quart and a half of water and strained in the fibers of the *Cyperus laevigata*. The liquid thus obtained is put into a container in which a medium-sized stone, heated red-hot, is placed. After boiling, the liquid is allowed to cool and, at the right temperature, it is taken internally. This is repeated until complete relaxation and sleep are fully restored. At the end, the scraped "iholena" or "lele" banana, thoroughly cooked in "ti"-leaves, is eaten. Spring water is used for regular drink. The young shoots of the "awa" are good for general debility, especially in children. Take the bud and chew it with the "ilima" flowers (about four of them) and give the mixture to the child morning and evening. This mixture is suitable for babies ten days old.

Again: For a workingman "awa" has proven to be a great healer for weary muscles and a great restorer of strength. Five mouthfuls of "awa" in a container mixed with about a cocoanut and a half of cocoanut milk, is strained and left in a container ready for drinking. The workingman takes a bath in a spring and returns ready for supper. Before eating he takes the drink of the prepared "awa" and then eats his supper. When he goes to bed he is ready then to enjoy a sound and dreamless slumber. In the morning he takes his spring water bath, eats his breakfast, and starts off to his work with renewed vigor and spirit.

For chills and hard colds, take the "awa" and have it chopped to bits that will fill about a hatful. Pound these roughly and soak in about a quart of water. At the same time, take about a quart of mountain apple buds and leaves; the outside of one green "kukui" nut; twenty "kookoolau" (*Campylotheca* spp.) buds and flowers, and the inside of one segment of white sugar-cane. Pound these together thoroughly and strain the juice coming from the mixture. Then put into it four heated stones, to cook it. This done, the liquid is allowed to cool to the right temperature. About a tablespoonful is then taken internally three times a day for three or four days in succession.

For difficulty in passing urine, prepare the "awa" as usual—five mouthfuls to a dose. Add to it four bits of the *Curcuma louza*, thoroughly ground to powder and about half or a little more of matured cocoanut milk. Cook the entire contents with a red-hot stone. In stirring the liquid, use five "ti"-shoots, one at a time, using only the tip of each shoot while stirring. When it cools to the right temperature the entire content is taken internally, followed by the eating of half of a sweet potato (either a "huamoa" or "mohihi") about the size of the fist—half of it being cooked and the other half to be eaten raw. Should constipation ensue, a proper laxative, in sufficient amount, should be employed. Three doses of this remedy are considered sufficient to effect a cure. A liberal quantity of spring water should be taken regularly during the treatment.

"Awa" root, in small quantity at a time, chewed every half-hour for three to five successive days, should bring about a cure for sharp, blinding headache. Move the bowels with salt water at the end of the treatment. The use of the "awa" in this fashion enables the individual to bar off contagious diseases of all sorts, especially skin diseases and eye troubles.

Ashes of "awa" are good for a child having general weakness of the body or for one having disorderly stomach and having thick white coating on the tongue. Take the ground-up left-over of the awa already used and burn it to ashes. Then add to it the ashes of the "pili"-grass and that of one "kukui"-nut thoroughly burnt. Mix the three kinds of ashes together and rub the tongue and lips and other afflicted parts of the mouth of the child with it three times a day for five successive days. For regular drink, the child should be given the "kookoolau" or the *Campylotheca* spp. tea.

For lung and kindred troubles take a hatful of the pieces taken from the main body of the "awa" and some of its partly dried roots; an equal amount of the *Portulaca oleracea* grass; four *Morinda citrifolia* fruits (fully matured ones); a hatful of the mountain apple buds and one piece of its bark the size of the palm of the hand. Have all these pounded together thoroughly and mixed in about a quart of water. Strain the water from this mixture and have it boiled or cooked with heated stones. After being cooled down to the right temperature, take about a pint of it at a time for three times a day and for five successive days. Should the remedy be too bitter for the patient, he may take a day off and during that time a new supply may be prepared for the next application. The remedy is generally known by the name "piipiiolono."

With the exception of the "awa-lau-ane-kane" (no scientific name given) "awa" is good for weaknesses arising from certain conditions during virginity. Take about a quart of the pieces coming from the main portion of the "awa" and four young "ti"-shoots. Pound these thoroughly and mix in about a quart of spring water. Have the whole strained and taken internally before meals morning and evening for eight successive days. After each dose, spring water may be taken to wash down the remedy and keep the mouth free from its taste and effect. Salty foods and fish with dark flesh should not be eaten during the treatment.

For displacement of the womb, "awa" has been found to be very helpful. Take four pieces of the meaty portion of the "awa"; a handful of "popolo" berries; four buds and two young leaves of the *Euphorbia multiformis* ("akoko"); two buds of the "kikawaioa" and a handful of the young shoots of the *Panicum pruricus* grass. Have these pounded together thoroughly and add to the mixture about two tablespoonfuls of the young cocoanut milk. Then have the entire mixture strained and the water derived from it put into a container ready for use. Before drinking it, chew and swallow about eight *sida* flowers. This prepares the way for the remedy to go in and, a little while after drinking it, half of a young cocoanut's milk may be taken in to clear the mouth of the taste of the remedy. This is taken morning and evening for five successive times. Take considerable spring water and *Campylotheca* spp. tea. This remedy is good for girls twelve years of age.

The different kinds of "awa" may be listed as follows:

(1) "Awa-hiwa": The leaves are somewhat round, smooth and shiny. It is dark; its segments are long and it is very frequently used by sorcerers in their medical practices. The young shoots and the roots are most useful as medicine.

(2) "Awa-moi": The general appearance of this "awa" is dark. The leaves are shiny and its segments are shorter than those of the "awa-hiwa." The joints are somewhat whitish in color. The young shoots are largely employed as medicine.

(3) "Awa-papa-eleele": In appearance, this resembles the former. Its segments are considerably shorter, however, and it grows wildly, its branches scattering here and there among shrubs.

(4) "Awa-keokeo": This "awa" is whitish in general appearance and is more commonly found than the others.

(5) "Awa-makea": This is white and has long segments like those of the "awa-hiwa" with reddish color at the joints.

(6) "Awa-nene" or "awa-kuaea": This "awa" is somewhat spotted with lumpy appearance of the bark and trunk. In general appearance, the spots resemble those of the turtle's back.

(7) "Awa-mokihana": The leaves are like those of the "awa-makea." Its segments are short and stubby. Its odor is somewhat fragrant, hence the name "mokihana," the famous fragrant berry of Kauai. It is a very powerful drink. It is sometimes called "Ka awa kau laau" because the birds take its bark and fruit to their nests.

8. "Awa-lauane-a-kane": This tree resembles in every way the "ulei" (*Osteomeles*). Its fragrant flowers are whitish yellow; its leaves are somewhat thick, having a disagreeable odor. As a medicine it has very small value. It is used chiefly as a poultice for boils. To prepare it, take two of its roots; two "pukamole" roots; one piece of the *Sadleria cyathecides* bark; a medium-sized piece of "kukui" bark and have these thoroughly pounded together. Then place the mixture in the fibers of the cocoanut and press out the juice. The liquid thus obtained is rubbed around the boil, leaving the eye untouched. The patient then exposes the boil to the heat of the sun to cause contraction as the sun dries the liquid around it. This application is made three or four times a day.

36. AWAPUHI KUAHIWI. (*Zingiber zerumbet*)

This plant grows wildly among the mountains of Hawaii nei. It is succulent and has long oval leaves that grow around the stem by enveloping it. Its flowers are yellow and very fragrant, growing in bunches, the juice from which the ancient Hawaiians frequently used for hair dressing.

The ashes of the leaves, mixed with the ashes of small leaf bamboo and these with the juice from four young "kukui" nuts make a splendid remedy for cuts and skin sores. The roots or bulbs of the "awapuhi" pounded with salt make helpful medicine for headaches. In applying rub the juice over the afflicted parts of the head.

For toothache take a bit of the root and have it partly cooked by rolling it over the coal fire. Shape it to fit the hollow of the troublesome tooth or the hollow caused by rot. Then bite it and leave it pressed for a while. As it becomes somewhat fixed in place, open the mouth and let the saliva flow. A single application may be all that is necessary should relief follow immediately   Otherwise the treatment should be repeated.

For ring-worm or for white blotches about the face, take two roots the the size of the forefinger, two *Cassis occidentalis* roots and have these pounded together with four pickings of Hawaiian salt.   Then add about a tablespoonful of child's urine to the mixture.   Strain the mixture and use the liquid from it for rubbing over the afflicted part of the face.   Apply this three times a day until cured.

For itch and kindred afflictions of the skin, leave out the urine and use in its stead two *Tephrosia piscatoria* roots.

For massage, take about ten bunches of the "awapuhi" flowers just about to open; four roots the size of the thumb; about a quart full of the buds of the sandalwood and a quart full of the *Tephrosia piscatoria*.   First, have the "awapuhi" roots and the buds of the sandalwood and *Tephrosia piscatoria* thoroughly pounded together.   Then drip into the mixture the water collected in the "awapuhi" flower bunches.   The entire mixture is then strained and the masseur, before beginning to massage, dips his hands into the liquid thus obtained, and rubs it over the parts to be massaged. This is done as often as the masseur requires to keep smooth the rubbing over the body, and to keep the skin from being bruised.   The application is made morning and evening for ten days.

For slight sprain or bruise, the "awapuhi" has been found to be very helpful.   Take eight roots the size of the thumb; two "awa" roots of equal size; one leaf of the *Chunbago zeylanica* and one fully matured *Morinda citrifolia* fruit.   Have these thoroughly pounded together and add to the mixture about a tablespoonful of water.   The whole is then mixed and the juice obtained therefrom is strained and put into a container.   The afflicted part is then bathed with it and massaged.   This is done morning ,noon, and before retiring.

37. AWAPUHI KEOKEO. (No specimen.)

The general appearance of this plant is like that of the "Awapuhi kuahiwi" except the size and height, which are smaller and shorter.   The flower, which is white, is very fragrant and it is wholly used for making wreaths.   Both the flower and root are used for fetid nostrils.   In preparing, take five flowers and have them withered in the sun.   Then have a handful of the sandalwood dust that is dried and two roots of the "awapuhi" the size of the thumb.   Crush the flowers and the roots together until thoroughly mixed and put the mixture in about a pint of water, with two heated stones, of medium size, to cook the entire content.   This done, the two stones are removed and the sandalwood dust is sprinkled into the cooked liquid.

After being thoroughly mixed, the whole is taken out and left to cool in the dew all night, thus conditioning the medicine for use.   The next day, a medium-sized ball of gauze is dipped into the liquid and the patient, taking it to the nostrils, inhales the odor and fume coming from it.   This constitutes the first treatment.   In the second treatment a tablespoonful of the "ti"-root juice should be added to the mixture before applying.   The application is made three or four times a day for five or ten consecutive days. At the end the patient takes a salt-water bath (at noon when the water is warm) three times a week, floating on his back and allowing the salt water to wash through his nostrils.   The mild salt-water laxative should be taken for internal cleaning.

38. AWEOWEO. (*Chenepodium sandwicheum*)

This plant resembles the "ilima" in general appearance and of somewhat reddish color.   It is a low-growing plant and is usually found in dry localities.   This remedy is good for general weakness in children.   For children that have a tendency to become weak, physically, the following applications are made:

(1)   For children five days old, four thoroughly chewed buds (flowers just beginning to open) are given for them to swallow.

(2)   For those three months old, six to eight buds, prepared in the same manner, are given.

(3)   From three months to one year, ten to twelve buds are given and the same amount is given till the children are two years old.

For beautifying the skin the preparation is similar to that of the "alani kuahiwi," which has already been described.   In addition, the mother, at the time when the offspring is about four months old, regularly chews the bark of the "aweoweo."   This is done once a day and at noon.   The amount of the bark to be chewed is about a pintful.   Together with it, "kukui"-nut, the fragrant seaweed "lipoa," and the bitter portion of the shell fish called "pupu-awa" are eaten by the mother.   The child receives all this through the mother's milk.

Again: The bark, sometimes, is pounded with water and the juice strained and mixed with the "lehua-poi," which the mother takes as food. All this is to effect beautification of the skin of the offspring during its growth and development.

For fattening or for adding weight, it was customary for the rulers and subjects of old to mix the potato with the "aweoweo" juice, with the following additions: The young shoots of the wild fern commonly called "uluhe"; "alaula," seaweed; shell fish, the bitter portion of the "pupu-awa"; and "ilima" flowers.   All these, in equal proportion, are thoroughly pounded together and the juice separated and strained.   Then it is mixed with either poi or mashed sweet potato and fed to the children.

39.   A-WIKI-WIKI.   (*Canavalia galeata*)

This plant is like a vine in its growth, and thrives in damp localities, especially in valleys having abundance of water or moisture.   Its leaves are flat and the flowers are red.   It is somewhat similar to the "aa-lii-kumakani."

The entire plant is used as a remedy for the itch, for ringworm and kindred skin diseases.   In preparing it, take a hatful of the leaves and the young shoots of the "awikiwiki" together with two pieces of its bark (the portion that is near the ground) the size of the palm of the hand and an equal amount of the mountain apple bark.   Add to this the entire *Cassia occidentalis* plant.   Have these thoroughly pounded together and then add about a quart of water to the pulp for mixing.   This done, the liquid from the mixture is strained and cooked with four medium-sized red-hot stones. The liquid is then allowed to cool to the right temperature and the patient is given a bath with it two times a day for five consecutive days.

40.   I-I.   (No specimen for identification.)

This plant is very much like the tree-fern ("hapuu") in general appearance with this exception, however, that it is smaller in size, and that the hairy substance growing around its stem is much more silky than that of the hapuu.

This plant is used as a remedy for raw sores over the body or for chafed skin.   To prepare it, take about a tablespoonful of the thoroughly dried silky substance that comes from the plant and mix it with an equal amount of the *Cyperus laevigata* fiber dust (thoroughly dried).   Add to this the juice of four young "kukui" nuts and then rub the sore or sores with the mixture.   Treat the patient three times a day.   For chafed skin leave out the "kukui"-nut juice and apply the other substances in dry and powdered condition two times a day.

For asthma (the kind that doesn't like the wind, as well as the dry cough asthma) the "ii" has been found to be very helpful.   Take four stems (free from the fine silky hairs), including the young shoots at the end.   Add to this four pieces (the size of the palm fo the hand) of mountain apple bark that are close to the ground; about a quart of the *Euphorbia multiformis* leaves; a hatful of the stems and flowers of the *Peperomia;*

about a quart of the stems, leaves and buds of the sandalwood; a piece of "kukui" bark the size of the palm of the hand, and one segment of the red sugar-cane "honuaula." Have these materials thoroughly pounded together and mixed with a quart of water, and then have the juice therefrom strained and cleaned. Then put into it a large-sized red-hot stone for cooking it. After it is cooked, it is allowed to cool to the right temperature and then the patient takes a mouthful of it at a time and three times a day.

Also, the "ii" is very helpful in removing foul breath and in stopping a tendency to vomit. Take the "ii" stem, scrape off the outside until the inside is wholly exposed, especially the central portion; then take a portion of it the size of the forefinger and pound it with the "hua-moa" sweet potato (the size of the fist). Add to this mixture the scraping of sufficient size of "ti" stem with about a quart of water. The liquid derived from the mixture is then strained and cleaned. The patient then takes the entire quantity. The result will be vomiting. As this takes place, the patient should make every effort to encourage it, thus removing from the stomach all causes giving rise to the awful feeling.

41. IEIE. (*Freycinetia arnotti*)

This plant grows like a vine or creeper. In general appearance its leaves and stem resemble those of the *Pandanus*. It creeps at great length over trees, and is found in abundance in the mountains especially where there is considerable moisture, rain or water.

For general debility giving rise to the white coating of the tongue, take eight stems of the "ieie" shoots, four medium-sized branches with flowers of the "kukui," one mountain apple bark the size of the palm, a handful of the *Peperomia* stems, the bark of the *Waltheria americana* tap-roots (two in number) and two segments of the white sugar-cane. Have all these pounded together thoroughly and the juice pressed out into a container to be strained and cleaned. Then the patient takes of the juice about a table-spoonful at a time for three times a day. For children a month old, half that quantity is given and for two times a day only. As the medicine grows bitter, especially at the end of about four days, a new supply should be secured.

For monthly periods of women where excessive discharge is experienced, take a lump of red clay the size of a "kukui"-nut and put it in a pint of water; a lump of grayish clay of equal size and put it into an equal amount of water and then allow the two lumps to dissolve separately. Then take four young stems of the "ieie" and have them scraped and cleaned; about a quart of the flowers, buds and leaves of the *Peperomia*, and a piece of "kukui" bark the size of an orange leaf. Have these pounded together and have the juice of the same pressed out and strained. By this time the two lumps of clay are either dissolved or softened to a watery state. The two are then thoroughly mixed and poured into the "ieie" mixture. The patient then drinks the entire contents and finishes by chewing a segment of the white sugar-cane. Salty foods should not be taken during the treatment, which usually takes five successive days to complete. Dark flesh fish also should be avoided. For drink, the patient should use *Campylotheca* tea during the entire period, and for a laxative, the *Impomea dissecta*.

For severe pain about the body, accompanied by high fever, the following is found most helpful: Take enough of the "ieie" shoots and leaves to cover a single bed. Then take two large *Alocasia macrorrhiza* leaves and have their ribs removed. These are then laid over the sheet with their faces up and over them are scattered the young shoots and the leaves of the "ieie." The patient then removes his clothes and lies down on this bedding of leaves in a naked condition. Over him is placed sufficient covering to bring about perspiration.

42. EKAHA KUAHIWI. (*Asplenium nidus*)

This plant is widely scattered among the mountains of Hawaii nei. They, like birds' nests, locate themselves at the fork of the branches of trees with their large blade-like leaves spreading out and down from all sides.

The use of this plant as a remedy has been found very effective for the general weakness of the body which gives rise to the heavy white coating on the tongue. In preparing it, take four of its young shoots (the very young leaves), twenty "lehua" buds or very young shoots; two pieces (the size of the palm of the hand) of mountain apple bark; one bark, of equal size, of the *Peperomia;* a medium-sized onion bulb, and two segments of the white sugar-cane. Have all these materials thoroughly pounded together and have the juice of the same pressed out and strained. In making the application, give one tablespoonful of the liquid thus obtained to children from three to six months old twice a day, morning and evening; a similar amount to those from seven months to one year old and two tablespoonfuls to adult persons. After taking the remedy, a piece of dried cocoanut may be taken to aid in neutralizing the taste in the mouth.

The juice derived from a mixture of twenty young shoots of "ekaha," two branches of "kukui" flowers, and two thoroughly roasted "kukui" nuts, all of which are thoroughly pounded together and mixed with the milk or juice of two young "kukui" nuts is most effective for sores about the mouths of young children from ten days to two years old. The juice is spread over the sores or about the mouth in case the child is troubled with heavy white coating on the tongue. The treatment is given twice a day for five successive days.

For ulcers or scrofulous sores about the body, the following mixture is found helpful: Eight "ieie" leaves with ribs removed; the bark of four *Cassia occidentalis* roots and about a tablespoonful of salt. Thoroughly pound these materials together and have the juice of the same pressed out and strained. Then, take the juice of one segment of sugar-cane that is derived by chewing and mix it with the other. The whole is then put into a cocoanut fiber container and gradually the juice is pressed out and into the opening of the sore or sores about the patient's body. The patient should bear the stinging effect of this remedy calmly. The application is made twice a day, morning and evening, for five times in succession.

43. EKAHA-KAHA. (No specimen.)

This plant resembles in every way the "ekaha" already given except it is smaller in size. It is used as a cure for asthma and for foul breath. Take four young shoots with four roots of the plant; a handful of "kohekohe" reeds (no scientific name given), two *Waltheria americana* roots (the bark only to be used), a good-sized *Morinda citrifolia* bark with two fully matured fruits and two segments of white sugar cane. Have these thoroughly pounded together and then have the juice from the mixture pressed out and strained. The patient then lays down with his face on the floor and drinks the liquid thus prepared. This is done twice a day for five successive days. For food, cooked fresh fish, "luau" and "popolo" leaves are good.

44. EKAHA-KU-MOANA. (No specimen.)

This is a certain growth in deep water where deep sea fish is sought. It grows like a tree and it is of coral make-up. A small piece from such a growth is used for sores about the mouths of children. The piece is ground to powder and mixed with the juice from the softening or partly decaying banana tree and from four young "kukui" nuts and a piece of mountain apple bark. The mixture is then applied directly to the afflicted part or parts of the mouth.

For lung trouble and for kindred diseases, the following mixture is found to be very effective: an equal amount each of the "koa," mountain apple and "kukui" bark (each piece being the size of the palm of the hand); about a quart full of the *Peperomia* stems and flowers; two onion bulbs; one partly dried cocoanut and two segments of the red sugar-cane. Have these materials thoroughly pounded together and then pour into the mixture the milk of a partly dried-up cocoanut. The liquid thus formed is then pressed out and strained. Then four medium-sized red-hot stones are dropped into the liquid to cook it. In the meantime, enough limbs of the "ekaha-ku-moana" have been gathered and powdered, producing an amount which would fill a tablespoon. This and an equal amount of the "ti" juice are then put together and poured into the above mixture after it is cooled to the right temperature. The entire content is then placed in a covered container where its strength can be conserved. The patient then takes about a tablespoonful of this liquid before each meal, morning, noon and at night. Salty articles of food and dark flesh fish should not be eaten by the patient. He should consume fresh fish cooked in "ti" leaves or broiled over the charcoal; also taro leaves, "popolo" leaves and other greens, after being thoroughly cooked. *Impomea dissecta* should be taken twice a week for laxative and *Campylotheca* tea for body-building.

45. IHI-AI. (*Portualaca oleraces*)

This is a creeping grass that thrives among the plains of Kahuku, Kawaihapai and Kaena, on Oahu. Another name for it is "lumaha'i," this being commonly known among the natives of Kauai. This remedy is largely employed to check the run-down condition owing to troubles about the vital organs. To prepare it, take a hatful of the plant; about a quartful of "ihimakole"; a hatful of the stems, flowers and young shoots of the *Peperomia;* the bark of eight *Waltheria americana* roots; the bark of eight "popolo" roots; the roots of eight *Sida* plants; eight *Pandanus* roots; four fully matured *Morinda citrifolia* fruits and four segments of the white sugar-cane. Have these materials thoroughly pounded together and then have the juice pressed out and strained. Into this liquid, pour about a tablespoonful of the burnt "ti" juice and, after being thoroughly mixed, the entire content may be placed in a covered container. A tablespoonful of this liquid is taken by the patient morning, noon and evening. Before using, however, the container should be well shaken. Avoid sour poi or potato, also fish with dark flesh. Eat heartily of the broiled or steamed white flesh fish, also bananas and cooked taro leaves and "kukui" nut. Use *Campylotheca* tea for drink.

46. ILIAHI. (Sandalwood.)

This grows extensively among the mountains of these islands. The leaves are somewhat round and are similar to those of the orange. The tree is like the orange tree, having smooth bark and very fragrant wood. The leaves share the same odor. The juice from its trunk is very bitter.

The sandalwood, as a remedy, is used for removing dandruff and for destroying lice. To prepare it, take a hatful of the sandalwood leaves; two pieces of the bark, and about a tablespoonful of the ashes of the dried "naio" wood. Pound the bark to pieces and crush the leaves and put the two into a container sufficiently filled with water. Then put into it two red-hot stones in order to heat the water and draw out the strength of the sandalwood. As the water cools down, the stones may be removed and the crushed bark and leaves taken out. The liquid thus obtained is then strained and t e "naio" ashes mixed with it. The mixture is then ready for use as a head wash. The patient dips his head into the container and, with his fingers, rubs the liquid into his scalp. This would kill the lice and destroy the dandruff. The application should be made three times a day,—morning, noon and evening, and for three days in succession.

For diseases of the sexual organs of both the male and the female, the "ili-ahi" has been used to advantage. The following preparation has been found most effective: Take five good-sized chewed "awa"-root balls and mix them in three cups of fully matured cocoanut milk. The liquid is then strained and put into another container. Into this liquid scatter about a tablespoonful of finely ground sandalwood, chili pepper, *Bobea*, and "kauila" wood. After mixing these thoroughly, the patient takes a mouthful of it at a time, morning and evening. At the end, the *Impomea dissecta* should be used as laxative for internal cleaning.

For the treatment of sores of long duration, the following preparation is recommended: Take about a quartful of the *Piper methysticum;* a piece of the *Jambosa malaecensia* bark the size of the palm of the hand, and have these thoroughly pounded together. Then add to the mixture about a quart of water and stirr the whole thoroughly. The liquid from this mixture is then strained and cleaned and placed into a separate container. Into this liquid scatter about a tablespoonful of each of these materials: the finely ground scrapings of the sandalwood, of the *Pelea cinerea* and of the *Bobea*. After being thoroughly mixed, the patient takes a drink of this every evening for five successive evenings. On the morning after the fifth time, a dose of *Impomea dissecta* should be taken for laxative, followed by the enema, using the slimy juice from the *Hibiscus tiliaceus* to remove all impurities from the lower bowels.

47. ILIEE. (*Chunbago zelanica*)

This vine grows abundantly among the plains and hillsides close to the seashore. Its leaves are long like those of the rice and it has yellowish flowers with seeds like peas. The juice of this plant is hot and, if mixed with salt, its effect is like the small chili pepper. For this reason it is good for swollen parts of the body. To prepare it take four of its roots about a quart of its leaves and an equal amount of its bark. Pound these materials together thoroughly with about a tablespoonful of salt. Then put the whole mixture into a cocoanut fiber bowl over which the milk from four young papaia fruits is dropped, endeavor being made to cover all of the outside of the porous container. This done, the medicine-filled fiber is passed over the swollen portion—a slight pressure with the thumb causing the liquid from the mixture to ooze out and spread over the skin. The constant application draws the matter (which causes the swelling) to the surface until it bursts out.

The "iliee" is also good for raw sores. Take about a quartful of the leaves and stems of the plant; an equal amount of the leaves and stems of the "la-ili" plant; and two vines (about an arm's length and about the size of the small finger) of the *Impomea dissecta*. Have these thoroughly dried in the sun and then pounded or ground to dust. Then take the milk from four medium-sized half-ripe papaia fruits and mix it with the dust to form a paste. In this condition, it is applied to the sore.

48. ILI-OHA.

This is the dark green moss which grows over rocks in streams and springs. It is good for sore lips or for sores which frequently appear at the corners of the mouth. Collect a handful of this moss and have it thoroughly dried in the sun. Then grind it to powder and apply it to the sore.

The "ili-oha" is also good for the burning within the chest. Take about a half of a quart of the moss and salt it with about a tablespoonful of Hawaiian salt. Then add to it the scraping of the "kika-wai-oa" stem and young shoot and about six thoroughly cooked young taro leaves. Have these well mixed before being eaten by the patient. In taking the medicine, have the patient lie down facing the floor. The medicine, then, is swallowed gradually, thus allowing it to do its work as it passes to the stomach. This is done twice a day for five successive times. After the treatment, the *Impomea dissecta* should be taken for laxative. The *Campylotheca* tea should be taken regularly by the patient during the treatment. Meat and salty foods must be avoided.

49. ILI-OHA LAAU. (*Erigen canadense*)

This tree resembles the *Morinda citrifolia*. Its leaves are somewhat yellow with reddish hue running through it, while its flowers are of yellowish white color. This remedy is good for sprain, backache and sore joints.

Take a hatful of its leaves; an equal amount of the "koa" leaves; about a tablespoonful of salt; a segment of the red sugar-cane. Have these materials thoroughly pounded together and placed in a cocoanut fiber container from which the juice is slowly pressed out and spread over the injured part. Slight massaging at the same time would help the patient.

This is done twice a day for five successive days. Spring water should be taken for regular drink.

For a fall or injuries caused by accident, the "ili-oha-laau" is found most helpful. Take about a quartful of the young shoots and leaves of the plant; a piece (the size of the palm of the hand) of the "kukui" bark; the bark of four "aumo-i" roots and about a tablespoonful of salt. Have these materials thoroughly pounded together and mixed with about a tablespoonful of the patient's urine. The entire mixture is then put into a cocoanut fiber contained from which the juice is pressed out and rubbed on the injury. Application is made twice a day for five successive times.

Again, take a hatful of its buds or young shoots and leaves; two pieces of its bark the size of the palm of the hand; a hatful of the young shoots or buds of the *Peperomia;* two pieces of the mountain apple bark the size of the palm of the hand; a handful of the "kohekohe" reeds which grow in taro patches; a handful of the dark water-cress; half of a partly dried cocoanut; two onion bulbs; two ripe and two green *Morinda citrifolia* fruits; and two segments of white sugar-cane. Have these thoroughly pounded together and then press the juice out into a separate container into which two red-hot stones are placed for cooking the liquid. After being thoroughly cooked, the liquid is strained and allowed to cool to the right temperature for drinking. The patient then lies down facing the floor with a cushion supporting his abdomen. About a pint of the liquid is taken at each time, this being in the morning, and only once a day, and for five successive times. A banana, called "iholena," is eaten after each dose. Dark-flesh fish, salty foods and meats should be avoided. Fresh white flesh fish cooked in "ti" leaves or broiled and young "popolo" leaves with "inamona" (cooked "kukui" nut) are good for food for the patient. The *Campylotheca* tea should be taken as a regular drink while the *Impomea dissecta* should be taken as a laxative after the treatment.

50. INIKO. (No scientific name given.)

This herb grows extensively on plains and pastures. Its leaves are like those of the tamarind tree, being finely pinnated. The pods are small and hard. Its sap is bitter. As a remedy it is good for rheumatic pain, for backache and for womb trouble.

To prepare it, take two whole plants of the "iniko," four "puakala" (no scientific name given) roots, two whole *Cassia occidentalis* plants and about a tablespoonful of salt. Have these materials thoroughly pounded together and then place the entire mixture in finely prepared cocoanut fiber bowl. With a slight pressure the juice from the mixture is forced out and allowed to spread over the afflicted part. By putting about a tablespoonful of this liquid into a half of a glass of water, the remedy may be taken internally. Such treatment, however, is usually given to cases having hard and dry cough.

51. ILIMA. (*Sida*)

The "ilima" is the plant from which the "ilima" wreath, a favorite of the Hawaiians, is obtained. Its leaves are somewhat round and its flowers are of yellowish color. As a remedy, the flowers of the "ilima" are most useful. For babies five days old, give four flowers (buds just opening), thoroughly chewed by the mother. For one from ten to thirty days old, give eight thoroughly chewed flowers, and from one to three months about twelve or more flowers. For older children, the hibiscus buds take the place of the "ilima." The "ilima" and the hibiscus flowers make very helpful laxatives for children, being mild and suitable to children's taste. While this treatment is being given the mother should take papaia and pork soup,—the young papaia fruit, finely chopped, being boiled with a small chunk of pork fat.

For womb trouble (especially when falling) the "ilima" mixture is very helpful. Take forty "ilima" flowers; an equal amount of the flowers and young shoots of the "popolo," and a piece of dry cocoanut. Have these thoroughly chewed and placed in a very fine piece of porous cloth. Then press out about a tablespoonful of the juice from the mixture and leave it to one side. The patient then places the enclosed mixture into her vagina as far in as is possible to place it. If this is done in the morning, the mixture is left there until noon, when it is replaced by a fresh one. As this is being done, the juice that is extracted from it is rubbed over the lower abdomen as near to the womb as possible. The treatment should be taken three times a day. The patient should not eat sour or salty foods. She should drink spring water or *Campylotheca* tea and should consume a certain amount of the "lele," "maoli" and "popoulu" bananas, also potato.

For general debility, the following mixture is effective: the bark of eight "ilima" roots; a handful of the young shoots and flowers of the *Waltheria americana;* about an equal amount of the flowers, the young shoots and stems of the *Peperomia;* a similar amount of the young leaves and shoots of the "popolo"; one fully matured *Morinda citrifolia* fruit; and two segments of white sugar-cane. Have these materials thoroughly pounded together and the juice pressed out and strained. Then take about a tablespoonful of the liquid three times a day. Have the patient take *Campylotheca* tea regularly and, at the close of the treatment, use *Argyreia tiliaefolia* for a laxative.

For asthma, take about a quart of the "ilima" flowers and young shoots; the bark of eight "ilima" roots; a handful of the *Psilotum triquetrum;* the bark of eight "popolo" roots; an equal amount of the "pukamole" roots; two segments of the red sugar-cane; and have these thoroughly pounded together. The juice from the mixture is then pressed out and strained. Two red-hot stones are then placed in the liquid to cook it; and, after being cooked, it is allowed to cool to the right temperature. The patient then lies down with his front to the floor while a cushion supports the lower portion of the abdomen. The medicine is then taken, the entire amount constituting one dose. The treatment is taken morning and evening for five successive times. *Capylotheca* tea should be taken regularly and the *Impomea dissecta* laxative at the end of the treatment. Sour poi and salty foods are prohibited.

52. ILIMA-KU-KULA. (No scientific name.)

This plant resembles the above in every way except that, because of its wild character and state, its leaves and flowers are much smaller than those of the cultivated "ilima." Its use as a remedy and the way it is prepared and applied are exactly the same as the other.

53. ILIMA-MAKA-NA-A. (No scientific name given.)

Again, this plant is, in every way, like the other "ilimas" except its leaves and flowers are much smaller than the second kind. Its use as a remedy is for dry skin—no perspiration coming from the pores. It is prepared in the following manner: Take two whole plants of the "ilimamakanaa," and, after the dirt is removed and the roots cleaned, they are tapped in order to loosen the bark from the wood. The wood then is removed and thrown away and the rest set aside. Then add four *Cassia occidentalis* roots; the bark of four "pukamole" roots (the kind having large leaves); four fully matured *Morinda citrifolia* fruits; and one and a half segments of the white sugar-cane. Have all these materials thoroughly pounded together and put into a container into which a quart of water is poured. Mix these thoroughly together and then place in the mixture four red-hot stones. As the liquid begins to boil, the patient is given a steam bath by being heavily covered and the steam allowed to get all over the body. After this, the body is washed with the same liquid. He is then removed to his bed and there, with his face down, he is given roasted sweet potato and thoroughly cooked "kukui" nut to eat. The following morning he is given a dose of the *Impomea dissecta* for internal cleaning.

54. INA-LUA. (*Cardiosperonum malicacabum*)

Refer to "laau poniu," as this is the same thing.

55. INA. (Sea egg.)

The "ina" is found in holes of the coral reef along the shore. There are two kinds: the whitish gray and black. The egg, with the exception of a small area around the teeth, is covered with spines. As a remedy, the "ina" is helpful for general debility of the body. Take four of the gray kind and four of the dark. Remove the spines and then collect about a tablespoonful of the slimy liquid from the region of the teeth of all of the eggs. This is rubbed over the tongue and lips of the child (ten days old or more, even six months old). Again, take four dark eggs, remove their meat and mix it with roast potato and feed the mixture to the child (one about a month old). After five treatments, the child is given internal cleaning.

56. IPU AWAAWA. (*Cucurbita maxima*)

This is a vine from which the Hawaiian gourd is secured. Its leaves are large, thick and hairy and of round shape. It has yellow flowers and hard-shelled fruit, from which the ancient style of Hawaiian calabash is made. Its young shoot and the leaves close to it are very helpful in case of partial insanity due to lack of sleep. The patient takes these and eats them. This is followed by the chewing of a piece of dried cocoanut with sweet potato and a drink of water. This is done twice a day for five successive times. After the treatments, a whole day of rest is taken after which the patient, using the meat or scraping from the inside of two fully matured or thoroughly ripe fruits, takes internal bath to clean out his bowels and, with about a quart full of water, he is given an external bath.

For bad blotches on the skin the meat of fresh green fruit is found most effective. To prepare it, take the meat of two young gourds the size of a large *Morinda citrifolia* fruit and put it into about a quart full of water. After being thoroughly mixed the water from the mixture is strained and used for internal cleaning. In making the application the water is allowed to enter the bowels slowly, the patient lying on one side and then on the other with the region about the navel being gently shaken to allow complete distribution of the water in the intestines, thus aiding in the complete removal of all impurities from within the digestive system. For food, the patient should take roast taro leaves and "kukui" nut together with sweet potato.

Again, the "ipu awawa" is very helpful to fallen womb. Take the inside of a young fruit, say the size of the head; a quart full of the young shoots or buds; the panicum pruricus grass and about two pints of water. Before adding the water, have these materials thoroughly pounded together. After this, allow the pounded panicum grass to soak in the water until the water turns green. Then scrape into this water the meat from the fruit and allow it to soak. This done, the water is strained and cleaned. In the meantime, a small ball (the size of a "kukui" nut) of soft and smooth cotton is prepared. When the water is ready, soak the cotton ball in it and then have the patient pass it carefully into the vagina and up to the womb. The result will be a warming-up effect in the region of the womb. Should this take place, the cotton ball should be left alone inside for a while before being taken out. If the treatment is administered in the morning, the cotton ball should be removed about noon. Immediately after removing, the vagina should be washed or flushed with the milk of the young cocoanut. No sexual intercourse should be permitted for at least three days.

And, again: The interior of the "ipu awaawa" may be used for internal cleaning of the bowels. Take a fruit and cut off the top so that a medium-sized opening be left. Fill it with water and then add to the water a thoroughly ripe *Morinda citrifolia* fruit. Then place the whole thing outside in the dew over night. The next morning the water is drawn out, strained and cleaned. In this condition, it is ready for the syringe.

57. IPU-HAOLE. (Watermelon.)

The watermelon can be made into a very powerful laxative. This is done by taking a young fruit the size of a coconut and having it thoroughly cooked and mixed with about two pints of water. Then drop into the mixture the juice of four "kukui" nuts and four spoonful of *Euphorbia multiformis* milk. These are thoroughly mixed and strained. The patient then drinks the entire contents followed by the chewing of a segment of white sugar-cane and the eating of a banana. The remedy will cause vomiting and a thorough washing out of the bowels. These effects, however, can easily be stopped by taking a drink of fresh water followed by the eating of cooked taro leaves ("luau") and roast sweet potato.

(*Note*—At this point Mr. Akina describes the use of the watermelon by cheap and murderous "kahunas" for evil purposes and therefore the description has no value to the science of medicine.—A. A.)

58. IPU-PU. (Squash, common variety.)

The squash is good for rash. Take a young fruit the size of a cocoanut and one young *Alocasia nacrorrhiza* tuber about 8 or 10 inches long and about as thick across as the fist. Have these cooked thoroughly and cleaned. Then, while they are still warm, have them mashed up in a container and mixed with water. The solution is then strained and cleaned. The patient takes a sufficient quantity of this liquid twice a day. On the following morning, however, *Impomea dissecta* should be taken in order to keep the bowels clean before another dose of the medicine is taken. For regular drinks during the treatment, the *Campylotheca* tea should be used.

59. IWA. (No scientific name given.)

The "iwa" is a certain kind of a fern having long leaves with stiff petiole or leaf stalk,—this stalk being frequently used for hat-making. The young top of the leaves and the roots are good for curing a bad case of stomach trouble. Take twenty young tops of the leaves; four roots; forty young tops of the arrow-root leaves; two handfuls of taro patch rushes (bunches of small reeds); a handful of the *Peperomia* stems; a piece of mountain apple bark the size of the palm of the hand; two fully matured *Morinda citrifolia* fruits and two segments of the red sugar-cane. Have these thoroughly pounded together and the juice from the mixture strained and cleaned and cooked with two red-hot stones. This done, the patient lies down on the floor on his stomach with a cushion supporting his abdomen. He then takes a sufficient dose of the remedy by drinking it. This is done once a day and for five successive days. After this, the *Impomea dissecta* is taken to clean the bowels.

60. IWAIWA or ANALII. (*Asplenium pseudofalcatum*)

This is another type of fern which is much smaller than the former, and it thrives on mountainsides, caves and in other places where there is much moisture. The leaves are much smaller and are stiff. The petiole is reddish in color and looks very much like the small end of a cocoanut-leaf stalk, the kind the old Hawaiians used for making brooms. As a remedy, the "iwaiwa" is found to be most effective for skin troubles such as sores, as well as for sores about the mouth.

A handful of the leaves is taken and dried. This is burnt to ashes. The ashes are taken and mixed either with the juice of four young "kukui" nuts or with the milk of two green papaia fruits, after which it is spread over the sore spot.

61. IWA-IWA KAHAKAHA. (No scientific name given.)

The use of this herb is identically the same as that of the above, both as a remedy and as a hat-making material.

62. IWA-IWA. (Same as No. 60.)

Another use found for this herb is beauty remedy. It is largely used for children up to six months old. Take five handfuls of the leaves and have the material thoroughly pounded and placed in a container. A quart of water is then warmed with the heat of the sun. This done, the pounded material is put into the water and stirred, and then strained and cleaned. The child (usually the pet of the family) is then given a bath with this water.

63. OHAHAWAINUI. (*Clermontia arborescene*)

This herb grows extensively among the mountains of Hawaii nei. The flowers are yellowish like those of the yellow ginger and equally as fragrant. The fruit, like that of the "kukui," is good for eating, and is one of the principal articles of food for the mountain birds of old Hawaii.

The milk from this herb is very effective for bad and deep cuts. To prepare it take two tablespoonfuls of the milk; one of the breadfruit milk; and one of the *Cyperus laevigata* dust (finely ground fibers). Have these materials thoroughly mixed and then a sufficient amount of the mixture is put into the cut. This is done morning and evening until the wound is healed. But, before making the second application, the wound should be thoroughly washed with the following: The water taken from thoroughly boiled "aiea" (no scientific name); or the liquid from thoroughly cooked *Cassia occidentalis*. After the washing, the wound should be thoroughly dried before applying the remedy. During the treatment the *Impomea dissecta* should be taken to keep the system free from impurities.

For asthma, the following mixture is very effective: twenty half-ripe "ohawai" fruits; four green kukui nuts; four tubers of *Curcuma louza;* about a quart full of the young shoots of the *Punex gigauteus;* a piece of the mountain apple bark the size of the palm of the hand; a handful of the *Peperomia* stems; two segments of the red sugar-cane, and two fully matured *Morinda citrifolia* fruits.

Have these materials thoroughly pounded together and the juice pressed out and cleaned. This is then mixed with the juice of the "ti"-root and then poured into a container. A mouthful of this liquid is taken by the patient three times a day for five successive days. Salty foods and meat are prohibited during the treatment. The patient may take fresh poi, sweet potato, boiled or broiled fish, "kukui"-nut and "luau" (cooked taro leaves).

The "ohawai" is also very effective for restoring or producing milk in the dry breast of the mother. Take about a tablespoonful of the "ohawai" milk and have it thoroughly mixed with the juice of eight *Euphorbia* leaves thoroughly pounded together with a half of a partly dried cocoanut, and a half of a segment of the white sugar-cane. The juice, of course, should be thoroughly cleaned before mixing it with the "ohawai" milk. While this is being done, a sweet potato is cooked and, after peeling it, it is hollowed inside and into it the mixture is poured. The opening at the top is then closed, and, with the thumb and fingers, gentle pressure is applied on all sides of the potato, thus enabling the liquid inside of the hollow to soak into the potato. The potato, thus prepared, is then eaten by the patient. Should milk fail to appear, laxative should be taken for internal cleaning and this followed by taking a soup made of the papaia fruit (in sufficient quantity) and a piece of pork. These are thoroughly cooked in sufficient amount of water.

64. OHE LAULIILII. (Small leaf bamboo.)
(No specimen for identification)

This type of bamboo is good for ulcers and scrofulous sores over the skin. Take about a tablespoonful of the bamboo ashes and mix them with an equal amount of *Cyperus laevigata* powder, a similar amount of the "lama" (no scientific name) powder, the milk of two fully matured papaia and the milk of two green "kukui" nuts. Mix these materials thoroughly and apply the mixture over the sores.

A mixture of bamboo powder (about a tablespoonful in quantity) with about a couple of teaspoonsful of the "naio" powder is good for stomach ache, providing, however, that the pain is not caused by "evil spirits."

65. OHELO PAPA. (No specimen for identification.)

The "ohelo" grows most abundantly near the volcano on the Island of Hawaii. It is a low-growing plant, having somewhat thick leaves of reddish color with flowers of pink hue and berries somewhat the size of small grapes. As a remedy the "ohelo" has been found to be most helpful for acute pain of the stomach. Take about a quart of the young shoots, leaves and berries of the "ohelo"; an equal amount of the *Dioclear violacea* leaves, both young and old; the same amount of the *Punex gigauteus* leaves, both young and old; a bulb of medium size of the *Curcuma louza;* a fully matured *Morinda citrifolia* fruit and one and a half white sugar-cane segments. Have these thoroughly pounded together and the juice pressed out and strained with the *Cyperus laevigata* fibers. The patient then drinks this liquid, taking sufficient amount morning and evening for five successive days.

66. OHIA or OHIA-KUAHIWI-AI. (*Jambosa malaecensis*)

This is the mountain apple tree which grows most abundantly among the mountains of these islands. The fruit is very juicy, of pink color and is very refreshing. The leaves are large and oval in shape. The flowers are pink, having needle-like pistils. The leaves, buds, bark and roots are very useful as medicine. Its different uses as medicine are as follows:

a. For deep cuts: Take two pieces of the bark the size of the palm of the hand and pound them thoroughly with a handful of the Hawaiian salt. The mixture is then put into a bowl of the cocoanut fibers and the juice pressed out and into the cut. The patient must exercise absolute self-control as the liquid burns its way into the flesh and nerves.

b. For general debility and stomach weakness: Take two pieces of the bark the size of the palm of the hand; a hatful of the leaves and young shoots; four medium-sized branches of "kukui" flowers; about a quart of the flowers, young shoots and leaves of the "hinahina" (gray looking herb that grows on the beach); two onion bulbs; about a quart of the flowers, young shoots and leaves of the *Waltheria americana* and two segments of the red sugar-cane. Have these materials thoroughly pounded together and the juice pressed out and strained. And, then:

(1) For children of one to two months old, about a teaspoonful should be given about twice a day;

(2) For those from three months to one year old, about a tablespoonful should be given; and,

(3) For those above one year, a mouthful should be taken three times a day.

Salty foods are prohibited, also sour poi. Fresh fish cooked in "ti"-leaves, together with cooked taro leaves, "kukui" nut and sweet potato are helpful articles of food.

c. For bad breath and for sores about the mouth: Take the bark about the size of the palm of the hand; a handful of the leaves of the *Psilotum triquetrum* and a half of a segment of white sugar-cane. Have these thoroughly pounded together and then add to the mixture about a quart of water. The entire content is then stirred and thoroughly mixed and then the liquid from it removed, strained and put into a container.

The patient then takes about a mouthful of this liquid to rinse his mouth with, morning, noon and evening for five successive days . After rinsing, about a tablespoonful of the liquid is taken internally.

The bark of the "ohia" may be chewed after the mouth is partly healed. This would hasten the healing process, as it quickly removes scabs and causes vomiting which brings out the tough phlegm that abounds about the throat and lungs.

The *Campylotheca* tea should be freely used by the patient. Salty foods should be avoided. Fresh fish, broiled over the coals, and fresh poi are good articles of food for this treatment.

67. OHIA—OHIA-A-PANE; OHIA-HAMAU; LEHUA-HAMAU.
(*Metrosideros collins polym, glaberrima*)
(Flowering specimen much desired.)

This tree grows to considerable size and height in the mountains of the Hawaiian Islands. The bark is thick with buds and flowers of reddish hue. The leaves are like those of the "lehua." Because of the height of the tree it has become the frequent abode of the "apa-pane" birds, hence the name "ohia-a-pane," a name given by the ancient bird-catchers. The tree is also called "ohia" or "lehua-hamau." This is because of the peculiar odor which it emits through its bark or wood.

The flowers of this tree are good for aiding in childbirth. Take about a span of the "hau"-bark (*Hibiscus tiliaceus*) and about the size of the palm of the hand when spread over a surface. Scrape this to threads in order to remove the slimy substance from it. Have this slimy substance mixed with water of sufficient quantity and then put into it four "ohia-a-pane" flowers. These flowers are rubbed between the thumb and the forefinger until they mix with the "hau" liquid and, with the fine cocoanut fibers, the whole thing is strained and put into a container. At the time when the pain of childbirth is most severe, the patient then takes a mouthful of this liquid.

68. OHIA-AI.

For sores about the mouth and for the foul odor that comes from such sores, the "ohia-ai" is a good remedy. To prepare it, take a piece of the bark the size of the palm of the hand and from that section of the tree touching the ground; a handful of the *Psilotum triquetrum* leaves and a half of one segment of the white sugar-cane.

Have these materials thoroughly pounded together and placed in a container. Pour into it about a pint of water and stir the entire content until thoroughly mixed. The whole thing is then strained and emptied into another container.

The patient then takes a mouthful of this liquid morning, noon and evening, rinsing the mouth thoroughly, making sure that the sores are washed, and continuing this operation for five consecutive days. After each wash a little of the liquid may be swallowed. A bit of the bark may be chewed in order to make the treatment more effective and hasten the healing process. Sometimes this is done in order to cause vomiting, thus removng the impurities about the throat and bronchial tubes. The patient should drink freely of the *Campylotheca* spp. tea and refrain from salty foods. Fresh poi and cooked fresh fish are good articles of food.

Again: For the removal of general debility of the body, the "ohia" is good. Take two pieces of the bark the size of the palm of the hand; a hatful of the leaves and young buds; four branches of "kukui"-nut flowers; a quartful of the flowers, buds and leaves of the "hinahina" (no scientific name) that grows on the beach; two onion bulbs; about a quartful of the flowers, buds and leaves of the *Waltheria americana* and two segments of the red sugar-cane ("honuaula"). Have these materials thoroughly pounded together and then the juice thoroughly strained with the fine fibers of the *Cyperus laevigata*. The treatment may be conducted as follows:

1. For children from one to two months old, give about a tablespoonful of the liquid;
2. For those from three months to one year old, give double doses;
3. For those above a year old, a mouthful is taken each time.

These doses are given twice a day to those below a year old, and three times a day to those above. For food, fresh fish either broiled over the coals or cooked in "ti"-leaves; broiled taro leaves ("luau"); "kukui"-nut; sweet potato and fresh poi are recommended. Salty foods should be avoided.

And, again: For children afflicted with white coating of the tongue and having a tendency to become weak, take a hatful of the buds and another hatful of the "lama" (no scientific name given) leaves, buds and fruits. Have the two mixed and left in about a gallon of water over night.

The next morning have four thoroughly heated stones put into the container and left there until the entire content is cooked. Then it is allowed to cool before the leaves, etc., are removed. The tea formed from the mixture is then strained in the *Cyperus laevigata* fibers and mixed with the "lehua" or "owene" poi. The patient then feeds on this poi together with broiled "hinalea" fish, fragrant sea-weed, "kukui"-nut butter and bits of "awa." The *Campylotheca* spp. tea should be used regularly.

69. OKOLEOMAKILI or PAU-O-PALAE or WAHINE-O-MAO or PAU-O-HIIAKA. (*Vigna luta*)

This plant resembles the *Peperomia* spp. in general appearance and grows around salty grounds near the beach and where there is considerable heat. Like the above remedy, this herb is used for the treatment of those afflicted with general weakness of the body. To prepare it take four buds and flowers for children from ten to forty days; eight for those from fifty days to three months; twelve for those from four months to six; sixteen for those from six to twelve months and a like proportion for those above a year old. When the child is a year old the treatment is no longer required. The mother takes the buds and flowers and, after chewing them thoroughly, feeds the child with the mixture.

This herb is also useful for the relief of asthma. Take a hatful of the flowers, buds, leaves and the matured portion of the plant; a similar amount of the leaves, buds and flowers of the *Peperomia;* two pieces of the mountain apple bark the size of the palm of the hand; a similar size of the "kukui" bark; four tap roots of the *Waltheria americana;* two half-ripe *Morinda citrifolia* fruits; a handful of the leaves of the *Psilotum triquetrum* and two segments of the white sugar-cane. Have these materials thoroughly pounded together and the juice from the mixture squeezed out into a container where it is strained with the fibers of the *Cyperus laevigata* and cooked with heated rocks or stones. After being cooked, the patient, lying on the floor with his face down and his abdomen resting on a cushion, drinks the liquid as he would tea. This is done twice a day. Meat is prohibited; also sour poi. The *Campylotheca* tea should be taken regularly. The treatment is usually ended with a dose of laxative.

This remedy is also very effective in cases of boils and ruptured skin. Take about a quartful of the flowers, buds, leaves and chunks of the wood of the plant. Have these thoroughly pounded together and placed in gauze. The juice is then rubbed over the sores and, in case of a boil, around it, leaving the head or eye of the boil free. Laxative should be used during the treatment.

70. OLAPA or OLAPALAPA. (*Cheirodendron caudicchaudii*)

This tree resembles the "koa" in general appearance and size. It has a peculiarly strong odor. The leaves are similar to those of the "naio" tree, and perhaps a little longer. The "olapa" grows in abundance among the mountains of Hawaii nei. The wood is good fuel even in a green state.

This tree has bark which, if mixed with other remedies, is effective for a bad case of asthma. This remedy may be prepared as follows: Take the bark of four "olapa" roots; the bark of four *Waltheria americana* roots; the bark of four "popolo" roots; a piece of the "koa" bark; four *Morinda citrifolia* fruits; a hatful of the leaves, flowers and fruits of the "popolo"; two segments of the white sugar-cane.

Have these materials thoroughly pounded together and the juice pressed out and strained. The patient then takes a mouthful of the liquid each morning and evening. *Campylotheca* tea should be used regularly together with the *Psilotum triquetrum* as drinking water.

71. OLENA. (*Curcuma louza*)

This plant grows like the ginger although small in size. Mixed with the other remedies, it becomes very effective for any growth in the nostrils or for offensive odor from the nose.

To prepare it take four "olena" bulbs the size of the thumb; the same quantity of ginger bulbs; twenty ginger flowers; eight clusters of ginger flowers and a half-segment of white sugar-cane. Have the "olena" and ginger bulbs and the half-segment of white sugar-cane thoroughly pounded together and the juice squeezed out, cleaned and put into a container into which the water or juice from the clusters of ginger flowers is dripped. Having the liquids well mixed, a small ball of the fine hair-like substance from the tree fern (the "pulu" fern) is made and enveloped in a piece of tapa. Into this ball of "pulu" the mixed liquids are dropped little by little until thoroughly drenched. The patient then inhales the odor or fume from this ball for as much as ten times a day. The ball is drenched once a day and as many days as are required to effect a cure. Use the *Sadleria cyathecides* for a gargle; the *Campylotheca* for tea; the "pakainui" for the internal treatment and the *Impomea dissecta* for a laxative.

For a gargle, take a piece of the "ohia" bark; a piece of "kukui" bark; two branches of "kukui" flowers and a handful of the *Psilotum triquetrum* leaves. Have these materials thoroughly pounded together and the juice strained with the finely prepared fibers of the *Cyperus laevigata*. Then add to the liquid the milk of one fully matured cocoanut. Having these thoroughly mixed, the patient then gargles his throat morning and evening and takes about a tablespoonful of the liquid internally after gargling.

With the omission of the cocoanut milk, and using, in its stead, two fully matured fruits of the *Morinda citrifolia;* one segment and a half of white sugar cane and one dried cocoanut, this same mixture becomes very effective for the offensive odor from the nose. And, by adding about a table-spoonful of the bitter juice from burnt "ti"-root, it becomes very effective for internal application, taking a mouthful each morning, noon and evening. Avoid eating meat and salty foods. Fresh fish, taro leaves and "kukui" nut are good articles of food.

For cleansing the blood, take four "olena" bulbs; about a quart of the shoots; an equal amount of the *Punex gigauteus* leaves and shoots; a piece of the mountain apple bark; an equal amount of "koa" bark; a half of a segment of white sugar-cane. Have' these materials thoroughly pounded together and the juice strained. The patient then drinks this liquid twice a day.

72. OLEPE. (No scientific name given.)

This plant grows in cultivated fields where moisture is abundant. The shape of the leaves is somewhat round, resembling the appearance of an oyster, from which the plant derives its name. This plant is used as a cure for bad cases of ulcer.

Take two "olepe" plants; two *Cassia occidentalis* plants; three "ha'u-oi" (no scientific name given) plants and four fully matured *Morinda citrifolia* fruits. Have these materials thoroughly pounded together and put into a container into which is poured about three quarts of water. After mixing the contents with this water, submerge about eight thoroughly heated stones in the following manner: four stones at the start and after the heat is fully spent, take another four and put them into the liquid. After the heat of these stones is given off, the last set is put in and then the mouth of the container is tightly closed with a covering that does not allow the heat to escape. The whole thing then is allowed to stand until it cools. Then the liquid is removed and cleaned and applied as a wash for the ulcer. Immediately after washing, and after the sore is dried, the finely powdered *Cyperus laevigata* and "lama" (no scientific name given) are scattered over it.

73. OLIWA or OLIANA. (No scientific name given.)

The "oliwa" is good as a remedy for removing weaknesses of the body. Take the bark of eight "oliwa" roots; four pieces of the bark of the trunk of the tree; two pieces of the "aiea" bark the size of the palm of the hand. Have these thoroughly pounded together and placed in a container into which two quarts of water are poured and mixed with the medicine. Then four heated stones are put in and, as the steam rises, the patient goes under cover together with the container of boiling liquid, for a sweat bath. This is done three times a day. In the meantime the *Argyreia tiliaefolia* is taken for a laxative and the *Campylotheca* tea for a regular drink. For food, take cooked fresh fish, "kukui"-nut and fresh poi.

This remedy is also good for washing ulcers, skin diseases and bad cuts. The use of the finely powdered *Cyperus laevigata* after the wash should not be avoided, however, for this will help to encourage the immediate growth of flesh during the healing process.

74. UWALA. (*Impomea* potato. Sweet potato)

The sweet potato has numerous varieties, all of which have distinct names and uses. Those that are known as having medicinal values may be set forth as follows:

a. UWALA-HUA-MOA: The leaves are somewhat round; the vine is whitish and grows to considerable length; the outside of the bulb is white, while the color of the inside of the bulb resembles that of the yolk of an egg. This potato is good for aiding those afflicted with vomiting. Scrape off about a pintful of the potato meat and at the same time scrape off an equal amount of the meat of the "ti" stem. These are then put together and mixed with sufficient amount of water. The entire contents are then placed in the heat of the sun and, when it is warmed, the liquid is removed and strained. The patient then drinks the whole of it. With the aid of tickling the throat with a feather, vomiting is developed until the yellow substance from the stomach—the cause of the disagreeable experience—is wholly removed. Together with this may come other matters which are equally troublesome.

b. UWALA-KIHI. (No scientific name given.) This potato has long white leaves with red ribs. The vine is whitish and of the same color as the bulb. The inside of the bulb is yellow while the part under the skin is pinkish. The potato is sweet and very good for eating.

This variety of potato is good for the treatment of bad cases of asthma, the kind which compels the patient to sit up continuously. To prepare it, take one potato the size of the fist; two pieces of the mountain apple bark the size of the palm of the hand; a hatful of the "hinahina-ku-kahakai" (no scientific name given); the bark of two large *Waltheria americana* roots and one segment of red sugar-cane ("honuaula"—no scientific name given.) Have these materials thoroughly pounded together and the juice pressed out into a container and strained with the *Cyperus laevigata* fibers. Then put into the liquid two red-hot stones with which to cook it. This done, the medicine is left to cool by itself. At the proper temperature, the patient, lying down on his stomach with a cushion supporting his abdomen, drinks down the whole of it. This is done morning and evening for five successive days. Salty foods should be avoided, also meats. The *Campylotheca* tea should be taken regularly and, at the end, a dose of the *Impomea dissecta*, in order to cleanse the bowels.

c. UWALA MOHIHI. (No scientific name.) The bulb is red on the outside while the interior is almost golden in color. The food quality is excellent. The leaves are somewhat rounded while the vine is reddish and grows to considerable length here and there. This potato is not frequently used in the mixtures of other medicines and the only use made of it is in the cure of vomiting and constipation. It is also used for patients suffering from lack of sleep. To prepare it: Take a bulb the size of the fist; a taro ("piialii") bulb of equal size; two pieces of the *Hibiscus tiliaceus* bark and the inside to four "kikawaioa" (no scientific name) stems. Have these materials scraped and mixed in a container into which sufficient amount of water is poured. The entire content is then shaken together and strained with the finely prepared fibers of the *Cyperus laevigata*. The patient then drinks the whole of it and retires (the treatment being given at night). In the meantime, the stems of the fully matured *Morinda citrifolia* fruits are being secured. The next morning these are boiled for about a half-hour; and, after being cooled to the proper temperature, the tea from these stems are used with the aid of the enema for injection and the washing out of the bowels—the patient lying on his right while the first injection is being made; then on his left, and then on his back for the final injection.

d. UWALA PIKONUI. (No scientific name.) This potato resembles the "mohihi" in general appearance, differing only in the shape of the leaves, the "pikonui" having leaves somewhat elongated and the joints of the segments of the vine somewhat dark.

By mixing with the other remedies, this potato could be made very effective as a stimulant for vomiting. The purpose of such treatment is to remove the thick, tough phlegm from the stomach or from the chest.

To prepare the treatment, take a bulb the size of the fist and have the meat scraped in very fine condition. Then take two large "ti" leaves and scrape the front of them until the required or sufficient amount is secured. The potato and the "ti" scrapings are then thrown together and mixed with a sufficient amount of spring water. The mixture thus formed is then strained and the liquid therefrom put into a separate container. The patient then takes this liquid and drinks it down. This is followed by tickling the throat, thus helping to start vomiting without delay. Salty water is recommended for drinking and, for cleaning the bowels, the *Impomea dissecta*. Bananas should be eaten freely. Salty foods are prohibited.

e. UWALA PU. (No scientific name given.) The outside of this potato is white and its leaves are somewhat iike those of the "uwala-hua-moa." The inside is very much like the pumpkin and is very sweet. This kind of potato is employed for womb trouble, particularly the fallen womb. To prepare it take a bulb the size of the fist and remove the skin; then take about a quartful of the flowers, young shoots or buds and the leaves of the *Peperomia;* the same amount of the flowers, buds and leaves of the "hinahina-ku-kahakai"; eighty *Morinda citrifolia* flowers; an equal quantity of the matured *Psilotum* fruits; the meat of one green "kukui" nut and three segments of the white sugar-cane.

Thoroughly pound these materials together and the juice therefrom pressed out and strained with the *Cyperus laevigata* fibers. Mix about a tablespoonful of Hawaiian starch and pour it into the liquid. Then put into the mixture two medium-sized stones that are thoroughly heated. After allowing the liquid to cook and after cooling it to the right temperature the patient then drinks the whole of it. This constitutes one dose. Two doses should be taken, one in the morning and one in the evening and for five consecutive days. The patient should take the *Campylotheca* tea regularly and he should not take too much food.

f. UWALA PI-API-A. (No scientific name given.) This potato is like the "pikonui" in general appearance and has the same medicinal value, use and application.

g. UWALA MU-KO-I. (No scientific name.) The leaves are spread apart while the inside of the bulb is dark. Its medicinal value is like that of the "uwala-pu," so is its use and application.

h. UWALA-APO. (No scientific name.) The inside of this potato is somewhat dark and it resembles somewhat the "uwala kahalaonaipu." Its medicinal value, use and application are similar to those of the "uwala kawelo."

i. UWALA-KEWALO. (No scientific name.) The leaves of this potato are like those of the "uwala-pu." Its medicinal value, use and application are also alike.

j. UWALA-KAHALAONAIPU. (No scientific name.) The leaves of this potato are somewhat round and the vine dark. It is sweet like the "apo" potato. Its use as a medicine is like that of "uwala-huamoa."

k. UWALA-UAHIAPELE. (No scientific name given.) The leaves of this potato have the appearance of palm leaves, having points around them. The inside of the bulb is dark with lavender hue. This potato has occupied an important part in the different mixtures of different doctors.

l. UWALA-KALA. (No scientific name.) The leaves of this potato are similar to the "uwala-uahiapele" leaves. The inside of the bulb has color like that of the "uwala-apo." The young leaves are good for table use if cooked with pork. This article of food is very strengthening to children; and, if cooked with four young taro leaves, together with the secretion ·of four "kukui" nuts, it becomes a very helpful laxative, both for children and adults.

m. **UWALA-LEHUA.** (No scientific name.) The leaves of this potato are dark with a sort of reddish hue. The vine is reddish in color, so is the outside of the bulb. The inside of the bulb resembles that of the "mohihi" potato. This potato is used in different mixtures, especially in the treatment of asthma. Like other potatoes, the milk is very useful.

75. UHALOA. (*Waltheria americana*)

This herb grows in almost all localities in Hawaii. The leaves are thick and hairy and grayish in color. The buds are good for children, say ten days old. The treatment is very much like that of the "ilima" flowers. The bark of the roots of a fully matured plant is good for sore throat. The bark is chewed and the juice swallowed. This may be repeated three or four times or until cure is effected.

For those affected with chronic cases of asthma or with pulmonary complication, the use of the *Waltheria americana* is very helpful. Take a hatful of the leaves, buds, flowers and six dried leaves of the buds; the bark of four roots; two handsful of the *Peperomia* spp.; four "ti" flowers; about a quartful of the "kohekohe" (no scientific name given); eight roots of the *Pandanus odoratissimus;* a half of a dried cocoanut; four *Morinda citrifolia* fruits and three segments of the white sugar-cane.

Have these materials thoroughly pounded together and the juice therefrom pressed out and strained with the finely prepared fibers of the *Cyperus laevigata*. Into this liquid empty the juice of a fully ripe papaia. Then put into the container about two hot stones in order to cook the entire content. When the heat from the stones has entirely ceased, remove them and, at the right temperature, the patient, lying down flat on his chest, drinks the entire content. This constitutes one dose. This should be taken in the morning and for five successive days.

Fresh fish well cooked and partly sour poi together with cooked taro leaves, "kukui" nut and "popolo" are good articles of food for the patient. He should take the *Campylotheca* tea for drink and the *Impomea dissecta* for laxative.

Again: For one with a run-down condition, losing weight and having much asthma, the *Waltheria americana* is very helpful. Take the bark of twelve roots of the herb; about a quartful of the buds; about four of the leaves below the bud; the bark of twelve "popolo" roots; about a quartful of the leaves, buds and four leaves just below the "popolo" buds; a half of a fully matured cocoanut; four *Morinda citrifolia* fruits; two segments of the white sugar-cane.

Have these materials thoroughly pounded together and the juice pressed out and strained with the finely prepared fibers of the *Cyperus laevigata*. Then put into the liquid two heated stones in order to cook it. This done, the liquid is allowed to cool to the right temperature. The patient, then, lying flatly on his chest with a cushion supporting his abdomen, drinks the entire content. This is followed by eating "iholena" or "maoli" banana and then a mouthful of cocoanut milk. This dose is repeated morning and evening for five successive days. The patient should take the *Campylotheca* tea for drink and the *Impomea dissecta* for laxative. Meat and sour poi are strictly prohibited.

76. UHI-KEOKEO. (*Dioscorea*)

This climbing vine is in abundance among the mountains of the Hawaiian Islands. The leaves are somewhat round like the "awa" leaves; the fruits are either round or long and having the same size as the "kukui" nut. The bulbs are like the potato but rather long and very good for eating. As a remedy, this is very helpful for heated body and for excessive sweating (probably very high fever). Take a bulb and scrape it to bits and have the pulp in three-quarters of a quart of spring water and add to it the scrapings of four "kikawaioa." Have these thoroughly mixed and have the patient take the entire mixture for one dose. This is repeated morning and evening and for five successive days. Have the patient drink spring water regularly and, at the end, have him take the *Argyreia tiliaefolia* for a laxative. Banana ("iholena") should be eaten frequently as well as fresh poi, fish and the "kikawaioa."

77. UHI-ULA. (Scientific name lacking.)

The general appearance of this plant is very much like the above ("uhi-keokeo"), the only difference being in the color and degree of hardness—the former being white and hard, while the latter is red and nutty. This plant is used as a cure for constipation.

To prepare it take a piece the size of a finger-joint and have it finely scraped and placed in a container. Then scrape the "piialii" (no scientific name given) taro in the same manner and have the two mixed. Then scrape the inside of four "kikawaioa" (no scientific name given) stems and with this have one *Morinda citrifolia* fruit, one piece of mountain apple bark and a segment of white sugar-cane thoroughly pounded together. This done, have all the materials mixed in one container and the juice strained with the finely prepared fibers of the *Cyperus laevigata*. Then a hot stone is dropped into the liquid to cook it. After it is cooled to the right temperature, the patient then drinks the whole of it. This dose is taken only in the morning and for five consecutive days. During the treatment, the *Campylotheca* spp. is regularly taken and, at the end, a dose of the *Impomea dissecta* is applied for cleaning the bowels.

78. UHIUHI. (*Mezoneurum kauaiense.*)

This herb is scarce among the mountains of the Hawaiian Islands. It may be found on the slopes of Haleakala near Kanaio or at Kauai. The wood is black and hard, while the bark is tough. The bark and young leaves are good for purifying the blood.

The preparation of the herb is as follows: A hatful of the young leaves and buds; four pieces of the bark nearest the ground; the inside of the trunk of the fern tree (a piece of the trunk about eight inches long with the outside chipped off or pealed off with a knife); a piece of the "ti" root of similar size; two pieces of the breadfruit bark; the bark of four *Waltheria americana* roots and two and a half segments of white sugar-cane. Have these materials thoroughly pounded together and the juice therefrom strained with the finely prepared fibers of the *Cyperus laevigata*. Then put into the liquid thus prepared about a tablespoonful of the "ti" juice. The entire content is then stirred and taken by the patient. Have the patient drink it three times a day. Food of all kinds can be taken. The use of the *Campylotheca* as a regular drink should be had every day. At the end, laxative should be taken.

78. ULU. (*Artocarpus incisa*—Breadfruit)

The "ulu" or breadfruit is found in nearly all localities in the Hawaiian Islands. Its leaves are large and lobed, while its fruit develops to considerable size. The fruit, when cooked, is like bread and is eaten. Very frequently it is made into poi.

The milk from the tree, when mixed with the secretion of the *Cassia occidentalis* and the ashes of tobacco, is very effective for skin diseases and for boils. For cuts, scratches, scaly or cracked skin, the milk is very helpful. For bad ulcers, the mixture of a tablespoonful of the breadfruit milk, a similar amount of the fine dust of the *Cyperus laevigata*, and an equal amount of the fine dust of the "lama" wood has been found to be very healing. Sores about the mouth can be treated with this mixture.

79. ULEI. (*Osteomeles anthyllidifolia*)

This plant is a sort of a vine that grows in abundance near the mountains, and it can be found at Kula, Ulupalakua, Kanaio and Kaupo on the Island of Maui. It also grows on the other islands. The leaves are small and round, the flowers yellowish in color and the wood very hard. The seeds are small and somewhat grayish in color. This plant is used as a remedy for the cure of general debility of the body.

For a child six months old, take six buds and four seeds and have them chewed thoroughly before he takes the mixture. For a child of one or two years of age, give a dose of twelve buds and eight seeds. This remedy, being a laxative, loosens the bowels and removes all impurities. By taking about a quartful of the leaves, the bark of eight "ulei" roots and about a pint full of Hawaiian salt and having them thoroughly pounded together, this herb becomes a very effective remedy for deep cuts. The juice from the mixture, poured right into the cut, acts most powerfully in hastening the healing process.

80. HAA. (*Antidesma palvinatum*)

This plant grows among the swampy grounds of the mountains. The trunk is very hard and the wood is somewhat reddish in color. The portion nearest the center is whitish. The size to which this plant grows is almost like the mountain apple tree. The leaves are very large. Of late, the "haa" has become very, very scarce. The use of this plant as a remedy is for the cure of vomiting spells. All that is done in the way of preparation is to take the leaves (in sufficient quantity) and chew them thoroughly before swallowing. This is followed by a drink of water and four small lumps of Hawaiian starch.

The "haa" has also been proven to be a very effective wash for ulcers and scrofulous sores. Take two pieces of the bark; the same quantity of the *Bobea* bark; two of the *Sideroxylon* bark; one *Cassia occidentalis* plant. Have all these materials thoroughly pounded together and placed in a container (say ,a gallon) half full of water. The pulp is then mixed with the water and the liquid thus obtained strained with the *Cyperus laevigata* fibers. Two heated stones are afterward placed in the liquid to cook it. These, in time, are removed and the liquid is allowed to cool to the desired temperature. The wash is then ready for application. After the sores are washed, apply the breadfruit milk together with the finely powdered *Cyperus laevigata* fibers and the "lama" powder.

81. HAU-KAE-KAE. (*Hibiscus tiliaceus*)

The "hau" is most abundant in the Hawaiian Islands. It grows thickly and wildly, its branches stretching with heavy growth in all directions. Its bark and wood are whitish in color and its wood very soft. Its large, thick leaves are round. The slimy substance which comes from its bark or from the base of its flowers makes a very gentle but very effective laxative both for adults and children. Usually, however, the flowers, especially those just opening, are used for this purpose. The doses depend largely on the age of the patient and they may be served as follows: For children from three to forty days old, four buds are used; for children from fifty days to three months, eight buds are used; for child from four months to eight months, twelve buds are used; for children from nine months to one year or more, sixteen buds are used. After this period, the base of the hibiscus flower is used instead of the "hau" flowers.

Should the bark of the "hau" be used, the following process is employed: Take four pieces of the bark (say about a foot long and three inches wide) and have them scraped to threads before placing them in a container. Add about three pints of water and have the entire content stirred and the slimy substance of the "hau" removed from the fibers. The liquid thus formed is strained with the finely prepared fibers of the *Cyperus laevigata* and put into another container. Before bedtime, the patient drinks this liquid and then retires. In the early morning, take forty *Morinda citrifolia* fruits and crush them to bits in a container of sufficient size. Add to the bulk about two quarts and a half of water and mix the content thoroughly. Then put into the content about eight thoroughly heated stones with which to cook it. This done, the stones are removed and the liquid strained with cocoanut fibers and then allowed to cool to the desired temperature. The enema is then applied, using this liquid for the injection. In applying the enema, however, care should be exercised that the injection is made in this manner: First—After the patient lies on his left side, after a small amount is injected, he shifts his position and lies on his right, again taking a small amount. Then he lies flat on his back and takes the rest of the liquid or as much as he can hold. Second—In the next application of the enema, the patient begins with his right side, then his left, and then on his back. This process will insure thorough cleaning.

Again, the "hau" is very helpful for congested chest when the phlegm is tough, making it hard to cough. Take two good-sized pieces of the bark; the young stems or shoots of the "kikawaioa" (no scientific name given) and four young shoots of the "uwiuwi" (no scientific name given). Have these materials crushed in a container and mixed with about a quart and a half of spring water. Thus the slimy substance is removed from the fibers and mixed with the water. Then have the liquid thus formed strained and placed in another container. In the meantime, the bark of four *Waltheria americana* roots, together with the bark of the same number of "popolo" (no scientific name given) roots are being thoroughly pounded and put into the finely prepared fibers of the cocoanut. The juice from this mixture is then pressed out into the "hau" liquid and mixed. In this condition, the remedy is ready to be taken by the patient. After the treatment, the *Impomea dissecta* is taken for laxative while the *Campylotheca* tea is taken for a regular drink. Bananas in good quantity should be eaten; also fish and partly sour poi.

And again: The "hau" is very helpful for a mother when delivering a child. The bark may be taken and the inside of it scraped so as to secure the slimy substance that comes from it. This substance is mixed with about a pint or a little more of water and taken by the mother either before or between the occurrence of the pain accompanying childbirth. A little of this liquid may be rubbed over the opening of the vagina, but care should be exercised in having the liquid hold the same temperature as that part of the body, thus providing no chance for contracting cold.

Furthermore, the "hau" may be used for dry-throat. The patient may take four very young shoots or buds and chew them thoroughly before swallowing. This simple dose is repeated twice a day, morning and evening. In time, the phlegm will be softened and the region about the throat softened and relaxed.

82. HAU-A-U. (No scientific name given.)

This is very much like the "hau kaekae" already discussed above. Its wood, however, is harder and darker than the "hau-kaekae." The flower is somewhat reddish. The slimy substance from the bark of this tree, mixed with about a quart of water and with sufficient scrapings of cocoanut and warmed in the sun, makes an excellent hair shampoo. The hair is dipped into the liquid up to the scalp followed by vigorous rubbing on the latter. The hair is then dried in the sun until the bits of cocoanut meat fall off from it. The hair may be dressed after that time.

83. HAU-HELE. (*Hibiscus sp. n.*)

The leaves of this tree are similar to those of the "awa" and are large. The general appearance of the tree is rough. The flowers are yellow and dotted with small spots. The base of the flower is used as a laxative for children from ten days to two years of age. The doses may be apportioned as follows: For children from ten to twenty days old, provide four flowers; for children from thirty days to one year old, provide eight or more flowers. These are taken and the base removed and chewed by the mother. 'From her mouth the dose is transferred to the child. This is immediately followed by feeding the child with the milk. When the bowels move, no further doses are necessary.

The small seeds from the "hau-hele" are good for children having general weakness of the body. These may be chewed and swallowed.

84. HALA. *(Pandanus odoratissimus)*

The flower of this tree is used for children inclined to be constipated For those from ten to sixty days old, the mother may take eight flowers and, after removing the soft portion which is at the base of the flower, chews it and feeds the child with it. This is followed with milk either from her breast or from the bottle. The treatment should be given twice a day.

This tree is well known in Hawaii. It is rugged and grows very high, its branches spreading far apart in all directions. The leaves are long and lined with sharp spikes. These are frequently used in hat and mat making. The trunk rests on its tubular roots far above the ground and it is tough and very strong. The flowers come in large clusters enveloped with long white and very fragrant leaves. The fruit, which is made up of a large number of small bodies containing its seed, also comes in cluster form. These small bodies are very fragrant and because of this they are frequently called flowers.

For the children from sixty days to one year old or more, use from twelve to sixteen flowers in one dose, and for adults use as many as the individual may want.

The root of the "hala" is very helpful for mothers who are weakened because of giving birth to a large number of children. Take eight roots; a handful of *Hydrogotyle poltata;* a handful of small reeds, "kohekohe" (no scientific name given); a handful of the young "hala" shoots; a like amount of the *Peperomia* stems; a quartful of the "makole" (no scientific name given) bark; an equal amount of the young shoots, leaves and seeds of the "naio" (no scientific name given); one dried cocoanut; four branches of "kukui" flowers; two fully matured *Morinda citrifolia* fruits; two and a half segments of white sugar-cane; two segments of red sugar-cane and have all these materials thoroughly pounded together and placed in a container. The juice from this mixture is then pressed out and strained with the fibers of the *Cyperus laevigata*. Then submerge two thoroughly heated stones for heating the liquid. The patient then lies flat on her stomach with a cushion supporting her abdomen and drinks the dose. This is repeated twice a day and as long as necessary. At the end, the *Impomea dissecta* is taken for cleaning the bowels. During the treatment the *Campylotheca* tea is taken regularly.

A widely used dose, especially by those having the same ailment but who do not possess much knowledge of the Hawaiian remedies, is as follows: twenty roots of the *Waltheria americana;* twenty "hala" roots; five *Morinda citrifolia* fruits; twenty young "hala" shoots; twenty young *Cyperus laevigata* shoots; five to six segments of white sugar-cane and a handful of red clay. These are thoroughly pounded together and the juice pressed out and strained with the *Cyperus laevigata* fibers. This done, the liquid is left in the container and covered with the *Cyperus laevigata* fibers. Over this cover, two mouthfuls of cocoanut meat (taken from a partly dried cocoanut) are placed and, over these, another two of the sweet potato called the "mohihi." These are then enveloped with the *Cyperus laevigata* fibers and the juice squeezed out into the liquid below in the container. This done, four well-heated stones are put into the container to cook the content. The patient then takes a mouthful of the mixture thus prepared morning and evening for five consecutive days.

Another use for the "hala" roots is for the cure of those troubled with pain in the chest. The following is the mixture with which it is used: Twelve "hala" roots; about a quartful of the "pa-ihi" (no scientific name given); the bark of four *Waltheria americana* roots; the bark of four "po-polo" (no scientific name given) roots; about a quartful of the buds, flowers and a couple of leaves of the *Waltheria americana;* about a handful of the *Peperomia;* the bark (about the size of the palm of the hand) of the mountain apple; four fully matured *Morinda citrifolia* fruits and two segments of the white sugar-cane. Have these materials thoroughly pounded together and the juice therefrom squeezed out into a container. Two well-heated stones are then put in, in order to cook the liquid thus obtained; and, after cooking it, and after it is cooled to the right temperature, the patient takes about a pint of liquid morning and evening. At the end, the *Impomea dissecta* may be taken for a laxative and the *Campylotheca* tea for a regular drink. Salty foods, including sour poi, should be avoided by the patient. Fish, "luau" (cooked young taro leaves), bananas and other fresh articles of food may be freely eaten.

85. HALA-KAHIKI. (Pineapple.)

This well-known fruit is largely used for purifying the blood. Take half of the pineapple after the outside is removed; the bark of the *Bobea* (four pieces each the size of the palm of the hand); four *Curcoma louza* bulbs; a piece (medium thickness and about six inches long) of a tree fern with the outside removed. Have these materials thoroughly smashed or ground and then add about a quart of water to the mixture. The liquid derived from the mixture is then strained and cooked with eight red hot stones. After the liquid is cooled, the patient then takes a mouthful of it at a time, morning, noon and evening. In order to make the remedy stronger and more stimulating, a tablespoonful of alcohol might be added.

86. HALA-PEPE. (*Dracaena aurea*)

This plant is employed for the relief from chills, high fever and the like. Take twenty buds of this plant; four pieces of its bark; the bark of four *Waltheria americana* roots; the bark of four "popolo" roots; and a half of the white sugar-cane segment. Have these materials thoroughly smashed and grounded together, and then add about two quarts of water. The liquid thus formed is then cooked with six red-hot stones. This done, it is allowed to cool. It is then ready for the use of the patient. The regular dose is a tablespoonful four times a day. The bowels should be cleaned at the end of the treatment. During the treatment the *Campylotheca* tea should be regularly taken by the patient.

Again: The "hala-pepepe" is very helpful for lung trouble or for a bad case of asthma. The dose is as follows: Twelve "hala-pepe" leaves; four good-sized pieces of the bark; the bark of one root; two pieces of mountain apple bark; the bark of four *Waltheria americana;* the bark of four "popolo" roots; a handful of the *Peperomia* stems; two fully matured *Morinda citrifolia* fruits; two segments of the white sugar-cane; and a half of a matured cocoanut meat. Have these materials thoroughly pounded together and the juice from them pressed out and strained with the *Cyperus laevigata* fibers. Then a tablespoonful of this liquid is taken out to one side and mixed with a tablespoonful of the Hawaiian starch. The, rest of the liquid is then boiled with four red-hot stones. When the liquid is steaming hot, take about a pintful of it off and pour it into the starch mixture just prepared. When the starch is cooked, empty the whole thing back into the rest of the liquid and have the entire content thoroughly stirred. The whole thing is then allowed to cool and, when it reaches the right temperature, the patient, lying on his stomach with a cushion supporting his abdomen, drinks the whole of it. This is repeated morning and evening and for five consecutive days. At the end, the *Argyreia tiliaefolia* powder is taken for a laxative. During the treatment, brackish water should be frequently used by the patient.

87. HAPUE. (No scientific name given.)

This plant grows most abundantly among the mountains of Keanae going over to Kanaio, also at Iao, Maui; Palolo, Manoa, Halemano and Waoala on Oahu and Hanalei, Lumahai, Wainiha, Kalalau and Waialeale on Kauai. The general appearance of this plant is similar to the *Hibiscus tiliaceus*.

When mixed with the "maaloa" (no scientific name given) the "hapue" becomes very effective in removing constipation and the itch about the anus. The dose may be prepared as follows: A quart of the "hapue" flowers, buds, leaves and roots; a similar amount and mixture of the "maaloa"; a handful of the buds and leaves of the *Euphorbia multiformis* and one segment of the white sugar-cane. Have these materials thoroughly pounded together and empty into it about two pints of young cocoanut milk. The juice from the mixture is then strained with the fibers of the *Cyperus laevigata* and mixed with about a tablespoonful of the Hawaiian starch. The patient drinks down the whole thing. This is followed by eating cooked young taro leaves and baked sweet potato. Should the bowels move too freely, causing general weakness of the patient, a mouthful of fresh water should be taken or a cold bath. But a free discharge from the bowels should be allowed until all impurities are removed and the intestines or the entire alimentary canal are left perfectly clean.

88. HAPUU (*Cibatium whamissoi kaulf.*)

This is the tree fern which thrives among the mountains of these islands. The downy substance which gathers about the young shoots is used for pillows. The meat within the trunk is very helpful for the purification of the blood and for stimulating the appetite. The dose may be prepared as follows:

Peel off the rough exterior of the "hapuu" trunk and save a piece something like eight or ten inches long; add about four *Curcuma louza* bulbs and eight *Punex gigauteus* roots. Have these materials chopped and thoroughly dried on hot stones. When dried, have them powdered and put into a container into which a quart and a half of water is poured. The entire content is then cooked with six red-hot stones. After being cooked, the liquid is strained with cocoanut fibers and mixed with about a tablespoonful of the bitter "ti"-root juice. The entire content is then left in a container. At the required time, usually in the morning and in the afternoon, the whole thing is thoroughly shaken and then the patient takes a mouthful of it for a single dose. This is repeated as often as necessary.

Again: This remedy is very helpful for those who lose weight and who suffer from pain about the chest. The dose may be prepared thus: Use the same quantity of the meat of the trunk as in the former dose and a like amount or quantity of the *Sadleria cyathecides* meat; have these dried on hot stones and powdered. In the meantime, collect these materials together: Two pieces of "kukui" bark the size of the palm of the hand; two pieces of the mountain apple bark; a like amount of the *Bobea* bark; the bark of eight *Waltheria americana* roots; the bark of eight "popolo" roots; the bark of eight *Cassia occidentalis* roots; two *Morinda citrifolia* fruits and two segments of white sugar-cane.

Have these materials thoroughly pounded together and mix the pulp with a quart and a half of water and then have the juice therefrom strained with the *Cyperus laevigata* fibers. Then empty into this liquid the powder just prepared, also four red-hot stones with which to cook the entire content. Cover the container well so as to retain the heat until the whole thing is well cooked. The liquid is again strained with cocoanut fibers. This done, the patient takes about a tablespoonful of it morning, noon, and evening for five consecutive days. On the morning of the fourth day, however, laxative should be taken. Should there be a leftover of the medicine by this time, the patient may continue taking it. Salty foods should be avoided throughout, also meat.

For hardened muscles, nervousness and tired limbs, the very fine and downy hairs of the "hapuu" are very good for treatment. These fine hairs are burnt and the heat from them is applied on the afflicted part or parts of the body, much care being exercised not to scorch the skin of the patient.

89. HEI. (*Carica papaya*)

The papaya tree is watery and soft and grows to considerable size and height. The leaves are large and resemble those of the palm tree. The fruit is delicious. The milk from the papaya is very effective in hastening the healing process in case of deep cuts, etc. The preparation is as follows: A tablespoonful of the "kukui" juice; a similar amount of the papaya milk; a like amount of the breadfruit milk and a tablespoonful of finely ground *Cyperus laevigata* fibers. Have these thoroughly mixed and then apply the mixture to the wound. In the evening, the wound is washed with the *Cassia occidentalis* water, after being thoroughly boiled. The wash is prepared thus: two *Cassia occidentalis* plants chopped to pieces and thoroughly pounded in about a quart and a half of water and boiled with four red-hot stones.

Again: The papaya fruit is good for mothers having dry breasts. Take a good-sized fruit that is partly ripe and have the outside and seeds removed. Have the whole thing chopped to bits and put into a container Empty into the container about a quart and a half of water and then have the entire content cooked with red-hot stones. While cooking, put in a piece of pork of sufficient size. After the whole thing is thoroughly cooked, and, after it is cooled to the proper temperature, the patient drinks the papaya gravy and eats the pork with poi just as she would her regular meal. After this, she takes fish broth, cooked young taro leaves ("luau"), etc., and at the end a laxative for internal cleaning.

90. HO-A-WA. (*Pittostorum* spp.)

This tree has a very large trunk. The wood is very hard. The leaves are large, broad, flat and black. The bark and the milk from it are bitter. This tree is found in all of the mountains of all the islands. The wood of this tree is used for the treatment of scrofulous swelling about the neck. The following is the preparation for the use of this remedy: Take eight "hoawa" fruits and remove their meat into a container. Add to this the meat of four "kukui" nuts; a quartful of the leaves and roots of the odoriferous plant, and an equal amount of the leaves, bark and roots of the *Chunbago zeylanica* plant. Have these materials thoroughly pounded together and then pour into the mixture about a tablespoonful of the bitter "ti" juice. The entire bulk is then put into the finely prepared fibers of the cocoanut and the juice pressed out and strained. With this liquid, the swollen spot is massaged.

91. HO-I-O. (*Dilazium arnottii*)

This plant grows very much like the *Phegopteris*, the difference between them being in the young shoots, those of the *Phegopteris* being soft and tender while those of the other are somewhat tough. Both are eaten as articles of food. The use of the "hoio" as a remedy is similar to that of the *Phegopteris*.

The special use of the "hoio" is for bringing a boil to a head. The young shoot of the "hoio" is ground to powder and then mixed with the milk of four "kukui" nuts. This done, the mixture is applied to the boil by gently rubbing around it, leaving the eye or the point from which the pus comes untouched.

92. HO-LE-I. (*Ochorosia sandwicensis*)

This tree grows to an enormous size. The leaves are as large as those of the "kukui" tree but oblong in shape. The nut resembles that of the "kamani." The meat is very delicious and is used for the relief from general debility.

To prepare it, take the meat of eight nuts, twelve *Sida* flowers and eight *Morinda citrifolia* flowers and have these materials thoroughly chewed together and fed to the child no younger than twenty days.

The bark of the "holei" is good for sweat bath. Take four pieces of the bark and eight leaves and place them in a container already holding about a quart and a half of water. When the patient is ready, and is under cover, place in the container two red-hot stones; and ,as these lose their heat, remove them and have another two red-hot ones to take their place. Continue doing this until the treatment is over. The steam thus generated is sufficient to provide for all the sweat bath needed.

93. KAA or MAUU PUKAA. (*Cyperus* sp.)

This grass grows very much like the *Cyperus laevigata*. It grows in bunches. The leaves are long and somewhat round at the bottom. Its use as a remedy is for destroying aches all over the body.

To prepare it, take a hatful of the buds, leaves, and roots of the "kaa"; one whole plant of the *Cassia occidentalis* that has not gone to seed; and a whole plant of the *Desmodium uncinatum*. Have these materials thoroughly pounded together and put into a container having about two quarts of salt water. The whole thing is then stirred and the liquid strained and put into another container. Put into it about four red-hot stones and, after boiling the liquid, remove them and allow the liquid to cool to the temperature suitable for bathing. The patient then is given a bath with the liquid morning and evening for five consecutive days. Each preparation should provide for two baths. This form of treatment is called "malani."

Again, this remedy is good for those whose ailment is of long duration, thereby causing constitutional weakness and loss of weight. Take a hatful of the "pukaa" grass; a whole "pukamole" plant; a hatful of the young shoots of the "ahihi" plant and two pieces of the *Aleurites moluccana* the size of the palm of the hand.

Have these materials thoroughly pounded together and mixed in a container with about two quarts of water. This done, the liquid thus obtained is strained with the finely prepared fibers of the *Cyperus laevigata*. The patient then bathes himself with this liquid, taking a mouthful of it internally. After the bath, he is given cooked taro leaves ("luau") and roast potato for food. On the following day, laxative may be taken for internal cleaning.

94. KA-E-E. (*Mucuna gigantia*)

This plant resembles the *Impomea dissecta* in general appearance. The leaves are somewhat round and the fruit is reddish in color. The meat of the seeds is a very powerful laxative. Because of the powerful effect of such a laxative, the treatment is named "kukapihe," that is, the effect may result either in the restoration of health or in the destruction of life. But the special use of this remedy is for bad cases of constipation and impure blood.

The preparation is as follows: Take the fruit and divide in half. Take one-half and have the reddish covering removed. The meat is then pounded on a board. At the same time the meat of four *Aleurites moluccana* nuts is being chewed. The two are then mixed in about a quartful of salt water and the liquid from such a mixture strained with the finely prepared cocoanut fibers. This liquid is applied internally by injecting it with the enema.

Among the names given for this form of treatment these are commonly used: "Waiki" and "Waiki-a-ku-ka-pihe."

95. KAUILA or KAUWILA. (No scientific name given.)

The "kauila" is a tree which grows to considerable height and size. The leaves are round and large and they resemble those of the mountain apple. The wood, especially the central portion of it, is reddish in color if fully matured, otherwise it is whitish. The tree may be found at Kanaio, Maui, or at Puukapele, Kauai. This wood is largely employed for the removal of skin contraction owing to fear; for fainting spells and for being subjected to fear.

To prepare it, take the wood of the "kauila" and scrape enough of it to fill a tablespoon. Empty the dust into about a pint of water and stir the entire content until the wood-dust is soaked and the patient then drinks down about a mouthful of it, bathing his entire body with the remainder of the content. This treatment is applied three or four times a day. The patient should use only the spring water for drinking and the *Impomea dissecta* for a laxative at the end of the treatment. The food should not contain any sour or too salty substances. It should be nice and cool.

96. KAU-NO-A. (*Cassitha filiformis*)

This air plant thrives at localities near the beach. It grows and hangs over shrubs and presents a mass appearance as its growth thickens. The color is reddish yellow. There are two kinds of "kaunoa"; the "kaunoa pehu" (the red type) and the "kaunoa uli."

The "kaunoa" is used as a remedy for removing from the chest the thick phlegm which causes congestion. The following is the preparation for the medicine: Take a hatful of the *Cassitha filiformis;* a similar amount of the *Psilotum triquetrum* finely chopped, and eight very young shoots of the "la'i" plant (young "ti" leaves). Have these materials thoroughly pounded together and placed in a container having about a pintful of water. The whole thing is then mixed and the liquid thus obtained strained and taken internally by the patient. It may be necessary, after some delay, to tickle the throat with a feather in order to hasten vomiting. Vomiting should be encouraged in order to cleanse the chest of impurities. The *Campylotheca* tea should be taken regularly and, at the end of the treatment, the *Impomea dissecta* should be taken for a laxative.

Again: For a woman giving birth to a child, the use of the "kaunoa" is very helpful, especially in removing the blood from the womb. Take a quartful of the "kaunoa" and have it thoroughly pounded and mixed with about a half of a pint of water. The liquid from this mixture is strained and given to the woman to drink.

97. KOA (Kahilikolo) (Koa-ku-makua and Koa-ku-mauna). (*Acacia koa*)

This tree grows to an enormous size and thrives most luxuriantly in the interior of the mountains of Hawaii nei. This is the type of "koa" out of which canoes were made. The leaves are sickle-shaped and the wood is very hard and wavy and is of reddish hue. The bark is very coarse. The name "kahilikolo" is taken from the place on which the "koa" grows in abundance and which is near Kilauea, Kauai. Because the "koa" creeps like a vine, growing over trees and shrubs and the branches sending out roots as it grows on, it is hard to determine the point from which its growth starts. Hence the name, "kalihi," or growing here and there over other plants and trees; "kolo," to creep, or growing like a vine or creeping plant.

As a remedy, the "koa" is employed for the relief of those who are long laid up in sick bed. Enough leaves are secured to cover the entire area on which the sick person lies. These are evenly distributed and the patient lies on them. The heat that comes from the contact of the leaves and body will cause considerable sweating. This should be encouraged until the patient falls off to sleep, thus indicating a restful condition of the body. Of course, as the sweat appears, it should be wiped off. On awakening, the patient will ask for food. This is a good symptom, an indication of restored health. Food, as much as advisable, should be supplied him.

Again: For children from six months to one year old who are inclined to be physically weak, the ashes of the "koa" are very helpful. The following should be the mixture: A tablespoonful of the "koa" ashes; a like amount of the dried cocoanut ashes; the milk of four *Aleurites moluccana* nuts. Have these materials thoroughly mixed together and, with the forefinger, the mixture is applied to the interior of the mouth of the patient, rubbing it on the roof of the mouth and on the tongue. This is done morning and evening.

98. KOA-I-A. (No scientific name given.)

This tree is somewhat similar to the above "koa" ("koa ku makua"), but this is smaller and more bushy in general appearance. The leaves are much smaller and finer than those of the above "koa" and when crushed they give out a very pleasing odor. The tea made from the leaves of this "koa" makes a very good wash for diseased skin.

To prepare the tea, take about two hats filled with the leaves; four pieces of the bark the size of the palm of the hand; four *Cassia occidentalis* plants and four *Desmodium uncinatum* plants without seeds. Have all these materials thoroughly pounded together and put into a container having about two quarts of water. Into this container, put about eight red-hot stones.

As the steam arises the patient takes a steam bath, and, as the liquid cools to the right temperature, the patient washes his entire body with it. This treatment is given morning and evening for five consecutive days.

99. KALAKALAIOA. (*Caesalpinia bonducella*)

This thorny, vine-like shrub grows like the *Impomea dissecta*. The leaves are large and seeds look like lima beans, only larger. This plant is used as a laxative for those having constitutional debility. The preparation is as follows: For children twenty days old, take half of the meat of one bean, grind it thoroughly and have them take it twice a day before meals. For those from forty to eighty days, a whole bean is given. And for those one year old or more, two whole beans are given.

For purifying the blood and for clearing the chest of tough phlegm, the following preparation is recommended: Take eight "kalakalaioa" beans; a piece of the mountain apple bark of sufficient size; a half of the fully matured cocoanut meat; the bark of eight *Waltheria americana* roots; the bark of eight "puakala" roots; a handful of the *Peperomia* spp. stems, and two segments of the white sugar-cane, and have these materials thoroughly pounded together and the juice from this mixture thoroughly strained. The patient then takes a mouthful of the liquid for a single dose and repeats this twice a day.

100. KALAIPAHOA. (No scientific name given.)

This tree grows to considerable height and size. The leaves are similar to those of the *Morinda citrifolia*. The front of the leaves is dark and the back is somewhat reddish. The wood of the male tree is dark red, while that of the female is white. This tree is found in nearly all of the mountains of the Hawaiian Islands. The wood of the male tree is employed for the cure of ulcers, scrofulous sores and asthma. The preparation is as follows:

Scrape from the wood of both the male and the female tree about four tablespoonfuls of wood dust and empty the same into about three pints of water, using spring water entirely. Mix well and then have the patient take a mouthful of the liquid for one dose morning and evening.

101. KALO. (*Coloccasia antiquorum*)

There are many varieties of taro, but they all have the same medicinal value (according to Akina). The selection of any of these is a matter of individual preference. The following preparations are regularly used:

1. Take any taro and have the outside removed and the inside scraped into a container of about a pint capacity. Add to that amount the juice of two and a half segments of white sugar cane; the meat of one fully matured cocoanut and two ripe *Morinda citrifolia* fruits. Have these materials thoroughly pounded together and the juice from the mixture pressed out and put into a container. This is strained with the fibers of the *Cyperus laevigata*. The patient then drinks this liquid as a laxative. The dose is taken five times in succession. Should stronger action of the bowels be necessary, the meat of the *Mucuna gigantia* seed might be added to the liquid.

2. Take a "lauloa" taro bulb and fix it as before. Then drop into it the juice of four young *Aleurites moluccana* fruits. In the meantime, a half of a segment of white sugar-cane and a half of a fully matured cocoanut meat are being pounded together and the juice therefrom pressed out and strained with the fibers of the *Cyperus laevigata*. This juice is then mixed with the taro. In this condition it is ready to be taken by the patient. After drinking it, the patient takes the luau or baked young taro leaves or potato leaves together with roasted potato for food. This food combination, however, helps to stimulate the bowels to move quickly, thus considerably aiding the action of the medicine. The dose should be taken only in the morning and for five successive times.

102. KA-MANO-MANO. *(Cenchrus calyculatus)*

This plant grows very much like a vine. The entire plant is very tender. The leaves are somewhat dark, round and spreading. The milk from it is very bitter. This plant may be found at Kipahulu and Keanae, Maui. As a remedy, the "kamanomano" is very good for deep and rotting scrofulous sores and for fresh deep cuts. The following is the preparation for the remedy:

Take about a quartful of the young shoots, leaves and roots of *Cenchrus calyculatus;* a similar amount of the bark of four "puakala" roots and about a half of a pint of Hawaiian salt.

Have these materials thoroughly pounded together and placed in the fibers of the cocoanut. Then squeeze the juice out and into the sore or cut. A sharp, burning effect will be experienced by the patient but this is only for a few moments' duration. As has always been experienced, healing results immediately. This treatment is known by the name "kaa-wili-moe."

103. KAMOLELAUNUI or PUKAMOLELAUNUI. *(Jussiaea villosa)*

This plant grows in taro patches. It has elongated leaves and small yellow flowers. The seeds are very tiny. The seeds and the white pulpy or pithy substances of the roots of this plant are good for small cuts or scratches about the body of a child. The following is the preparation: Take the seeds and spread them on the scratch or sore as you would powder. These seeds will dry up the sore and clear the way for healing. Or, if the white substance is used, the application is made the same way: The white substance is spread over the sore as an absorbent and left there until noon, when it is removed to be replaced by a new one. This, again, is repeated in the evening, and as many times as necessary.

104. KAMOLELAULII or PUKAMOLELAULII. *(Polygonum glabrum)*

This plant grows very much like the above. The difference between the two being the size—the former being larger than the latter. The medicinal value of the two, however, is about the same. The use of the two plants is for purifying the blood. The following is the preparation:

Two *Polygonum glabrum* plants; two *Jussiaea villosa* plants; one piece of the tree-fern meat about fourteen inches long, thoroughly dried in the sun; four *Curcuma louza* bulbs; a like amount of the *Punex Gigauteus* bulbs and four bulbs of the darker *Curcuma louza*. Have these materials thoroughly pounded together and then add about a quart and a half of water. Drop into the mixture about four red-hot stones and then cover the opening of the container tightly and allow time to thoroughly cook the content. This done, the liquid is strained with the fibers of the cocoanut and put into a clean container. Then add to it the juice of one and a half white sugar cane segments. The patient then takes about two tablespoonsful of the liquid for a single dose and this is repeated three times a day morning, noon and evening, and as many times as the medicine lasts Salty foods are prohibited, also dark flesh fish. A dose of the *Impomea dissecta* should be taken every four days while the *Camplotheca* tea should be taken every day. The use of the cooked young taro leaves, potato leaves, "popolo," *Aleurites moluccana* nut meat, bananas, potatoes, *Dioscorea* bulbs, etc., is recommended.

105. KANAWAO ULAULA or PI-O-HIA or KUPUWAO.
(Broussaisa arguta and B. pelluoida)

This tree resembles the *Pandanus odoratissimus* in growth and in general appearance. Its color is of reddish hue. The leaves are rough, also the bark. The flowers are somewhat the same as the sunflower. The fruit, which is as large as a pheasant egg, is rough. The trunk is somewhat succulent in character.

The use of this tree as a remedy is for the purpose of building up the physical constitution of the body. But, according to the ancient belief, this remedy is for the purpose of bringing about conception with a barren woman. To prepare it, take a hatful of the "kanawao" fruits and, ten days before menstruation, the patient eats five "kanawao" fruits with two eggs that are baked in "ti"-leaves. Before eating, however, prayer must be made to the great Giver of all gifts for His special blessing. This treatment is for an adult woman.

For a younger woman desiring conception, two "kanawao" fruits should be eaten with baked eggs, repeating this for five successive days. When menstruation takes place, and after a couple of days flowing, sexual intercourse may be had, thus bringing about a conception of life.

For a mother whose children do not live, the dried "kanawao" fruits, regularly eaten from conception to the time when the child is old enough to feed himself, will remove such ill-effect.

106. KANAWAO-KEOKEO or PIOHIA. (*Cyrtandra* sp., white variety)

This tree resembles the *Broussaisa arguta* and *B. pelluoida* in general appearance except in size and color, this being larger, especially the leaves, and of white tinge. The fruit is in a cluster form and is used for the same purpose as the "kanawao-ula." In addition, however, the ripe fruit is used for those afflicted with weak physical constitution, both young and old people. The following is the preparation for this remedy: One ripe fruit constitutes one dose for children from ten to forty days old; two ripe fruits for those from fifty days to three months old; four ripe fruits for those from three months to six months old; and from six to eight ripe fruits for those from seven months to one year old. Above this age, the use of the fruits ceases and the treatment takes the form of regular drink (medicine not stated) every morning before breakfast.

107. KAWA'U. (*Styphelia tameiameia*)

This tree grows to considerable size and in abundance among the mountains of these islands. The trunk resembles the "ohia" tree, the *Jambosa malaecensis*, and the wood is very hard. In ancient days, this wood was frequently used for making "tapa" clubs. The bark is whitish in color, so is the wood. The flowers are large. The flowers are used for the cure of ulcers and bad scrofulous sores. The preparation is as follows:

Have twenty "kawa'u" flowers, a like amount of the *Cyperus laevigata* young shoots and about a tablespoonful of the "lama" scraping or dust thoroughly dried out in the sun. These are then pounded together or ground into powder. This done, the powder is scattered over the sores of the patient and allowed to remain there until the scab, which forms there, dries and peels off. The *Impomea dissecta* should be taken for a laxative, spring water for drinking water and the tea made from the interior of the tree fern for a regular drink.

108. KI. (*Cordyline terminalis*)

This plant grows in abundance among the mountains of the Hawaiian Islands. The so-called "ki" refers to the trunk and roots of the plant, while the large oblong leaves are named "la'i." The flowers are in large clusters. The leaves are used for under-ground oven cover or for cooking fish or pork in, or for fishing drag. The root, when cooked, is very sweet and is used for food. When fermented, it becomes a very powerful alcohol. The "ki" flowers are used for a certain mixture for the cure of growth in the nose. The following is the preparation:

Take about two pints of the "ki" flowers; four *Curcuma louza* bulbs about the size of the thumb; four *Zingiber zerumbet* bulbs (the wild variety); four *Zerumbet* bulbs of the domestic variety. Have these materials thoroughly pounded together and the juice therefrom pressed out and strained with the fine fibers of the cocoanut. In the meantime, about a tablespoonful of the fine dust of the sandalwood and "naio" is being secured, and emptied into the "ki" mixture. This done, add to the whole about four tablespoonsful of water and stirr the entire content thoroughly. Then empty about a tablespoonful of the bitter juice of the "ki" into the whole thing, thus putting it into condition for use. A small ball of tree fern hairs is then made and soaked with the medicine. The patient, holding this ball before him, inhales the fume or odor that comes from the medicine. This he does vigorously for five or six times a day.

Again, the "ki" flowers are used for relieving asthma. Take eight "ki" flowers; two medium-sized chunks of the *Sadleria cyathecides* and *Asplenium nidus*, the outside of which being removed and the inside being thoroughly cooked in an underground oven. Have these materials thoroughly pounded together and the juice pressed out and cleaned. This juice is then mixed either with the potato or taro poi and taken by the patient. When this supply is exhausted, the next may be secured in the same manner. The patient should avoid cold foods. The baked young taro leaves and the mashed *Aleurites moluccana* nuts should be eaten and these should be taken in warm condition, with the *Campylotheca* tea for a regular drink to be taken four or five times a day.

For a severe case of asthma, the following preparation is recommended: Four "ki" flowers; eight very young "ki" leaves; a hatful of the *Peperomia* spp.; the bark of four *Waltheria americana* roots; a handful of the *Waltheria americana* flowers; four ripe *Morinda citrifolia* fruits; one *Impomea batatas;* and three segments of white sugar-cane. Have these materials thoroughly pounded together and the juice therefrom pressed out and' strained with the fibers of the *Cyperus laevigata*. The patient then takes a mouthful of the liquid and gargles with it. Then he takes another mouthful and swallows it. The dose is taken three times a day and as long as the supply of the medicine lasts. Following the treatment comes another which is made up of the following: Eight *Impomea dissecta* roots; one ripe *Morinda citrifolia* fruit; the bark of two *Sida* roots; and a handful of the white portion at the bottom of the young *Pandanus odoratissimua* shoot or very young leaf. Have these materials thoroughly pounded together and emptied into a container having about a pint of water. The entire content is then mixed and the liquid therefrom separated and strained with the fibers of the *Cypera laevigata*. This done, the yolk of an egg and a quarter of a tablespoonful of starch are dropped into the liquid and stirred thoroughly. In the meantime a chicken is being cooked and the broth from it made ready. The patient then takes the prepared liquid. As the bowels begin to move, the broth is taken in sufficient amount. This encourages passage of waste from the system. When the system is clean and there is no further need of the operation of the laxative, water or fresh water bath may be taken. Or, the patient's face may be sprinkled with cold water. These will stop the movement of the bowels.

Again: The "ki" leaves and the very young shoots are very helpful in removing the congestion of the chest and lungs owing to the tough phlegm which accumulates there. The following preparation is recommended: Eight young shoots of the "ki" and four leaves and one potato—*Impomea batatas*. These are carefully scraped and mixed in about a pint of water. The patient then drinks the whole dose at once. In some cases vomiting would start at once; and, in some, it would be necessary to tickle the throat. In either case, vomiting should be encouraged until the patient feels somewhat hollow about the chest, thus indicating a thorough cleaning out of the lungs. Brackish water should be taken five times a day. It is well to take a laxative after the treatment, followed by the enema and using the *Hibiscus tiliaceus* water for the injection.

Again: The leaves of the "ki" are very helpful for dry fever. By this is meant the burning heat of the body without sweating. The following is the method of preparation for the remedy: Take the "ki" leaves and have the ribs removed. These are then tied together in a belt form,—one leaf to another,—in order to get around the body. The head of the patient is then wrapped with one of these belts and so is his chest and abdomen. Once wrapped, the pores of the skin will open and the body will throw off its poison from the sweat glands. The patient, however, must take extreme care not to contract cold at this time. The treatment should be administered twice a day,—morning and before retiring, removing the "ki" leaves in the afternoon and in the morning of the next day. The relief to the patient comes after much sweat has been drawn out . It is always advisable to take laxative after the treatment and, during the treatment, to use the *Campylotheca* tea.

Again: The green and the ripe "ki" leaves finely combed and made into a wreath and worn as such, are very effective in providing restful condition of the nerves and body of those afflicted with a run-down physical health. The patient will have restful sleep, which is very necessary to the administering of treatments by a physician.

And, again: The following mixture of "ki" flowers and the young shoots is very effective for very bad cases of asthma. Take five "ki" flowers; twenty "ki" shoots; five handfuls of the *Peperomia* spp.; five handfuls of the "ihi-awa" (no scientific name given); twenty *Pandanus odoratissimus* roots; five handfuls of the leaves and very young buds of the "popolo"; twelve ripe *Morinda citrifolia* fruits; eight segments of white sugar-cane. Have these materials equally divided into five lots, thus making five doses for the patient. This done, the first lot is thoroughly pounded together and the juice therefrom pressed out and strained with the fibers of the *Cyperus laevigata*. A red-hot stone is then dropped into the liquid to cook it. After cooking it, and, after cooling it to the right temperature, the patient takes a drink of the whole of it. The next dose, taken in the evening of the same day, is prepared in the same way and so on until all the doses are taken out. In drinking it, the patient should lie on his stomach with a pillow supporting his abdomen. The doses are taken morning and evening.

109. KIHAPAI. (*Lochnera rosea*)

The leaves of this plant are thin, the flowers having white and sometimes reddish hue. The juice from it is very bitter. By mixing with the other remedies, an effective solution can be secured for purifying the blood. The mixture is as follows:

Take four pieces of its bark the size of the palm of the hand; a similar amount of the mountain apple bark; a hatful of the leaves, buds and stems of the *Peperomia* spp.; a like amount of another variety ("pohina") of the *Peperomia* spp.; four clusters of the *Aleurites moluccana* flowers; a half of the fully matured cocoanut; about a pintful of the "lehua" (red variety) flowers and four segments of the white sugar-cane.

Have all these materials thoroughly pounded together and the juice therefrom pressed out and cleaned with the fibers of the *Cyperus laevigata*. Drop into the liquid a couple of red-hot stones in order to cook it. After cooking it, cool it to the right temperature for drinking. The patient, then, lying down on his stomach with a pillow supporting his abdomen, drinks the whole of it. This dose is repeated twice a day and for five successive days. Salty foods are prohibited. Laxative should be taken at the end of the treatment. The *Campylotheca* tea is recommended as a regular drink.

110. KIKANIA. (*Desmodium uncinatum*)

This plant grows abundantly all over the Hawaiian Islands. Its leaves are coarse and round and it has burrs surrounding the seed vessels. The leaves, say eight at a time, when thoroughly dried in the sun, crushed to powder, put into a pipe and smoked by the patient like smoking tobacco, are very soothing, and, if a sufficient amount is taken four or five times a day, the patient would experience relief. This remedy is for the treatment of asthma.

When the "kikania" powder is mixed with the *Campylotheca* tea, and taken regularly by the patient, it becomes a very effective remedy for cold in the head or for general debility. And, like other treatments, a dose of the *Impomea dissecta* should be taken at the end for internal cleaning. And, should it be necessary to continue the treatment for some time, this laxative should be taken every four days.

Again: The "kikania," when mixed with other herbs, makes a very good wash and remedy for scrofulous sores, for boils and ulcers. The following combination is recommended: Take a whole "kikania" plant that has not gone to seed; four *Cassia occidentalis* plants; two "ha-u-oi" plants; two pieces of the *Bobea* plant. Have these plants finely chopped and mixed in about two quarts of water. The mixture is then thoroughly boiled with eight red-hot stones put into it. This done, the content is cooled to the right temperature and then the tea is strained with the fine cocoanut fibers. The sore is then washed and dried and, after this, it is covered with the mixture of equal parts of the *Cyperus laevigata* and "lama" powders. This treatment is repeated until the sore is healed. At the same time, the *Impomea dissecta* should regularly be taken for internal cleaning and the patient should use blood purifying remedy.

111. KOWALI AWA. (*Impomea insularis*)

This vine grows in abundance here and there in these islands. Its leaves resemble the palm of the hand and the flowers are somewhat whitish in color. The whole vine, from the flowers to the roots, makes excellent laxative. The following preparation is recommended:

Take twenty flowers and an equal number of the leaves and a piece of fully matured cocoanut meat. The latter is pounded thoroughly and then mixed with the "kowali" flowers and leaves, wrapped in the "ki" leaves and baked over the coals. After the mixture is cooked, the patient eats the whole of it. This is followed by drinking chicken broth, eating cooked fish and baked young taro leaves and roasted *Aleurites moluccana* nuts. The laxative will act immediately and it should be allowed to have free course until the bowels are thoroughly clean. The patient then takes the *Campylotheca* tea and bread. Should the bowels continue to move too freely after this, a mouthful of fresh water should be taken by the patient and this will stop the action of the laxative.

The flowers are also good for the general weakness of children. For those ten days old a couple of flowers are chewed and given to them by their mothers. This amount is steadily increased until the age of thirty days. Above this age, four flowers are used at a time for the treatment.

Again: The "kowali awa" is very helpful to those having severe backaches. Take a hatful of the flowers and leaves of the vine; twenty large vines the size of the forefinger and a half of a handful of Hawaiian salt. Have the materials thoroughly pounded together and pasted on the back where the pain is. This is held to its place by a wide piece of bandage wound around the body and over the medicine. This is repeated morning and evening, the patient going to bed with the medicine. The number of applications depends largely on the duration of the pain. Laxative should be taken by the patient twice a week.

Again: The "kowali awa" is very effective in the case of a broken bone. Take four large roots of the "kowali"; a hatful of the leaves of the "iniko"; eight "kowali awa" flowers; an equal amount of *Impomea dissecta* flowers; and about two pints of Hawaiian salt. Have these materials thoroughly pounded together and, after having the broken part of the bone properly adjusted, pour the juice from the mixture over the injured part and then put the whole bulk right over it. The medicine is held in its place by a wide piece of bandage wrapped and fastened around it. It is claimed that this treatment with this medicine far surpasses any other, the "kowali" being the most effective in knitting the severed parts of a broken bone as well as healing the flesh-wound around it. On the battlefields of olden days, the "kowali" was specially used for spear wounds and broken bones.

112. KOWALI PEHU. (*Impomea dissecta*)

This vine is very much like the former in appearance. There is a little difference, however, in the leaves of the two—those of this variety are somewhat round and thicker. The value of the two vines as medicine is the same.

This variety is largely used as a laxative. The preparation is as follows: Take six *Impomea dissecta* roots; one ripe *Morinda citrifolia* fruit; the bark of two *Sida* roots and one very young shoot of the *Pandanus odoratissimua*, especially the very white portion of it. Have all these materials thoroughly pounded together and placed in a container having about three pints of water. Have the whole content thoroughly stirred and the liquid thoroughly strained with the fibers of the *Cyperus laevigata*. Then a mixture of one egg and a tablespoonful of Hawaiian starch is dropped into the liquid and the entire content is then stirred until it is uniformly mixed. The patient then drinks the whole of it. In the meantime, chicken broth is being made ready, and this is taken in sufficient amount by the patient in order to hasten the action of the remedy and to continue such action until the system is thoroughly clean. When this is accomplished, and the patient no longer needs the action of the laxative, fresh water may be sprinkled on the face or it may be taken internally with a cold bath following.

113. KO. (Sugar cane.) (Many varieties.)

There are very many varieties of sugar cane, but those regularly used for medicinal purposes are the "ainakea; ko-kea" and the "honuaula," all of which have not been given their scientific names. The very young shoot of the cane is very effective for bad cuts. The preparation is as follows:

Take four very young shoots of the sugar cane; two *Impomea dissecta* vines of sufficient size and about two pints of Hawaiian salt. Have these materials thoroughly pounded together and put into a large piece of cloth and tied into a ball. This is wrapped with the "ki" leaves and baked over the charcoal. After it is cooked and cooled to the right temperature, the juice from it is squeezed out and directed into the cut. If any member of the body is entirely severed, the same could be restored to its place by placing it over where it has come off and, after having it fastened to its proper place with the aid of the dried banana stalk this furnishing a groove in which the injured part lies with the severed portion held in place and fibers, by pouring the liquid from the medicine over and around the cut. It is claimed that the strength of the remedy not only hastens the knitting of the severed parts but eliminates the scar from where the injury has occurred.

114. KOOKOOLAU. (*Campylotheca* spp.)

This herb grows in abundance among the mountains of the Hawaiian Islands. It is not very high. Its branches spread out in all directions; its leaves are somewhat rugged and its flowers are small and yellowish in color. As a remedy, it is very effective especially for general debility of the body.

For children from ten to forty days old, the mother may feed them with six flowers and buds thoroughly chewed. This is followed by feeding them with milk. Those from fifty days to eight months may be given the *Campylotheca tea*—eight leaves, buds and flowers broiled in about two quarts of water,—and the tea thus made taken as a regular drink. For the older children, the proportion may be increased to twelve leaves. For the adults, eight leaves may be boiled in about a quart and a half of water.

A mixture which is very helpful is as follows: Take two *Campylotheca* plants; the bark of four *Waltheria americana* roots; about a quartful of the buds, flowers and leaves of the *Waltheria americana;* the bark of the mountain apple the size of the palm of the hand; four medium-sized branches or clusters of the *Aleurites moluccana* flowers; a hatful of the *Peperomia;* two fully matured *Morinda citrifolia* fruits and two segments of the white sugarcane.

Have these materials thoroughly pounded together and the juice from the mixture pressed out and strained with the fibers of the *Cyperus laevigata*. The patient then takes a mouthful of this liquid three times a day. Banana (the "iholena" and "popoulu") should be eaten in sufficient quantity and the treatment should be followed by taking the *Impomea dissecta* laxative.

Again: The *campylotheca* is very helpful for throat and stomach trouble, also for stimulating the appetite. The following is the preparation:

Take a quartful of the flowers, buds and the leaves of the plant (either green or dried); a half of a quart of the seeds and buds of the *Psilotum triquetrum;* a quartful of the flowers and the buds of the *Waltheria ameri-*

cana; an equal amount of the young leaves of the "lehua" (the red variety) and a segment of the red sugar-cane.

Have these materials thoroughly pounded together and placed in a container holding about a gallon and a half of water. Place in the entire content about four red-hot stones and then cover the mouth of the container tightly. Allow the content sufficient time to get thoroughly cooked and then remove the cover and the stones and let it cool to the right temperature when it is put into the *Cyperus laevigata* fibers to strain the liquid that is to be used as medicine. This done, the patient takes a mouthful of it for one dose three times a day and for five successive days. This tea may be taken during meals with bread, taro or potato. In some instances, the buds and leaves are chewed together and the same result is acquired by the patient.

Again: For bad cases of asthma, the *Campylotheca* is very effective. The following mixture is recommended: Take a hatful of the flowers, buds and leaves of the *Campylotheca;* a handful of the seeds and leaves of the *Psilotum triquetrum;* double amount of the flowers, leaves and stems of the *Peperomia* spp.; a quartful of the flowers and the leaves of the other variety ("pohina") of the *Peperomia;* two pieces of the mountain apple bark the size of the palm of the hand; a quartful of the young leaves of the red "lehua"; four clusters of the *Aleurites moluccana* flowers; a burnt *Aleurites moluccana* nut; a half of a fully matured cocoanut meat; four ripe *Morinda citrifolia* fruits; four segments of the white sugar-cane and a quartful of the *Potulaca oleracea.* Have all these materials thoroughly pounded together and the juice therefrom pressed out and strained with the fibers of the *Cyperus laevigata.* Then cook the liquid with two red-hot stones. This done, the liquid is cooled to the right temperature and then the patient, lying on his stomach with a pillow under his abdomen, drinks the whole of it. This constitutes one dose. This is repeated in the evening of the same day. The next morning, the same thing is done and this is continued for five successive days. Salty foods should be avoided. The laxative, *Impomea dissecta,* should be taken at the end of the treatment, while the *Campylotheca* tea is taken regularly during the treatment. The banana ("iholena" or "maoli"), cooked fresh fish and the baked *Aleurites moluccana* nut meat are good articles of food for this treatment.

115. KOKIO or PUAALOALO. (*Hibiscus*)

This plant is very much the same as the foreign hibiscus introduced into the islands. There are two varieties and these are known by their flowers. The one is of a reddish color and the other is yellowish. The medicinal value of both is the same. The leaves and the buds are largely used for softening the contents of the stomach and bowels, especially in cases of constipation.

For children, the bottom of the buds are chewed and fed to them by their mothers. For the adults, the young leaves are chewed and swallowed. The slimy juice that comes from the leaves or from the buds acts as a gentle laxative for the system and is very helpful for general debility and for a run-down condition.

For purifying the blood, the following preparation is recommended: Take eight pieces of the root of the hibiscus; four pieces of the *Bobea* spp. bark the size of the palm of the hand; a similar amount of the mountain apple bark; the bark of eight *Waltheria americana* roots; one *Desmodium uncinatum* plant without the burrs; four *Impomea Pescaprae* roots; two pieces of the tree fern (*Cibatium vhamissoi kaulf.*) that are partly dried; two *Cassia occidentalis* plants; four matured *Morinda citrifolia* fruits; a segment and a half of the red sugar-cane.

Have all these materials thoroughly pounded together and put into a container having about a quart of water. The whole thing is then cooked with about six red-hot stones; and, after having it cooked, the content is emptied into the fibers of the *Cyperus laevigata* and the juice pressed out and strained and left in a separate container. The patient then takes a mouthful of the liquid three times a day before meals and for five successive days. Together with the doses, the *Campylotheca* tea should be taken regularly and all salty foods avoided. At the end, the *Impomea dissecta* should be taken to effect thorough cleaning of the system.

116. KOLI ULAULA and KOLI KEOKEO. (*Ricinus communis*)

The appearance of these two plants is the same, the only difference being in their color,—one being red and the other white. As remedies, both have equal values. They are usually applied to cases of severe headache and fever. The following is the preparation:

In the case of a child having strong fever, the "koli" (either red or white) leaves are gathered in sufficient quantity and these are put around its head (leaving the top part) and around its body with something wrapped around the leaves to hold them in place. This done, the cover, either a heavy sheet or a blanket, is put over the child. The leaves then will draw the perspiration out as the heat of the body increases. Sweating should be allowed to freely take its course since relief is sure to follow the elimination of the poison from the system.

For adults, the same course is followed.

117. KUAWA. (*Psidium guayava*)

The guava grows most abundantly anywhere in the islands. The tree spreads its branches considerably and, in rich soil, it grows to considerable height and extent. The leaves are oval and somewhat rough. The flowers are small and white. As a remedy, the guava serves as an effective agent for deep cuts, sprains and other injuries, largely due to accidents, in a wonderful way. Take a quartful of the buds of the guava; a similar amount of the buds and leaves of the *Tephrosia piscatoria;* twenty very young cocoanut leaves; two handfuls of the flowers and buds of the "hau-oi"; two pints of Hawaiian salt and a half of a segment of the white sugar-cane. Have all these materials thoroughly pounded together and placed in the fibers of the cocoanut. The juice from the mixture is then squeezed out and on the injured part, the patient bearing the burning effect with much self-control, especially in a case of a bad cut. But once the remedy covers the injury, the healing becomes thorough in its process.

Applied to diarrhoea, the guava buds and the Hawaiian starch mixed are very helpful agents. For children from two to six months, six buds thoroughly chewed by their mothers and given to them, followed by the feeding of about eight small lumps of Hawaiian starch, will stop the looseness of the bowels. And, for adults, the dose is increased to twelve buds and twelve medium-sized lumps of Hawaiian starch. Should the diarrhoea continue, another dose may be taken. And, should it still continue, then a laxative must be had followed by the enema. The slimy juice of the *Hibiscus tiliaceus* extracted at night by placing sufficient number of the very young shoots in the water, is good both as a laxative and as an injection. Or, the liquid from forty fruits of the *Morinda citrifolia* boiled in about two quarts of water may be used for the enema.

Another use of the guava is checking hemorrhage of the bowels or of the intestines. Take three guava roots; two *Pandanus odoratissimus* shoots (the young white portion); and a handful of the Chinese banana roots. Have these materials thoroughly pounded together and put into a container having about a gallon of water. Into the container, place about four red-hot stones and then have the opening of the container covered tightly. After the content is cooked, have the stones removed and the liquid strained with the fibers of the *Cyperus laevigata*. The patient then takes a mouthful of this liquid for a single dose. If that does not stop the hemorrhage, another dose may be taken, and perhaps another until the trouble is checked. At this point, the patient stops using the medicine. Onions and salty foods should be avoided during the treatment.

118. KUKAEPUAA. (*Panicum pruricus*)

This grass grows in abundance anywhere in these islands. The leaves are long and hairy. The edge of the leaves are sickle-like in that it cuts. This grass is used as a remedy for those having a run-down condition.

The following is the preparation: Pluck about sixteen very young shoots (young leaves) and have them thoroughly chewed with a piece of fully matured cocoanut meat. And, for very young babies, this mixture is fed to them by their mothers, followed by the feeding of milk from the breast. For a laxative, only the grass is chewed and fed to the children. This will remove from the system the filth which caused the general weakness of the body.

For adult patients, the young shoots of the grass may be chewed and swallowed and this is repeated three or four times a day.

For the hemorrhage of the stomach and bowels, take a sufficient amount of the grass to fill about a quart and then have it thoroughly pounded. After being pounded, add about two quarts of water and have the whole thing thoroughly mixed and the liquid from it strained with the fibers of the *Cyperus laevigata*. This done, the patient then drinks the whole of the liquid; and, after a little while, he eats about one "iholena" banana, a half of it at a time. Then he takes about a tablespoonful of raw Hawaiian starch thoroughly mixed with water. This dose is repeated as long as necessary. When the hemorrhage stops, the patient stops taking the medicine.

Another use of the grass is for the cure of the cataract in the eye. Twenty very young shoots are thoroughly chewed or reduced to the consistency of a thick liquid. This is blown into the eye right where the cataract has grown. This is repeated morning and evening for five successive days. At the end, the patient washes his eyes with clean water and this is repeated each morning for five successive days. Salty foods should be avoided. The patient should consume only those articles of food that are fresh and thoroughly cooked. Sour poi should not be eaten. As a regular drink, the *Campylotheca* tea should be taken. Laxative must be had at the end of the treatment.

119. KUKUI. (*Aleurites moluccana*)

This tree grows most abundantly among the mountains of the Hawaiian islands. The leaves are toothed and flat and have yellowish gray color. The flowers come in clusters. They are small and whitish in color. The nuts, like the flowers, also come in clusters. They are round and have very thick covering of grayish color. The nut itself, imbedded within the thick cover, has very hard shell within which is the white and rich meat which is eaten as food. When cooked, it is called "inamona." In its raw state it is called "kukui."

The entire tree is very useful. Aside from the wood which is used for fuel, the flowers, nuts and bark make very effective remedies for the removal of very many weaknesses of the body caused by the stomach and bowels. The following are the preparations made for specific troubles mentioned in connection with them:

For children from six months to one or two years old who are affected with general weakness of the body due to stomach or bowel disorder, this mixture is recommended: Four clusters of "kukui" flowers; two handsful of the *Peperomia* spp. stems without leaves; two pieces of the bark of the *Jambosa malaecensis* the size of the palm of the hand; one thoroughly baked "kukui" nut; one onion bulb; one fully matured fruit of the *Morinda citrifolia;* two segments of the white sugar-cane.

Have all these materials thoroughly pounded together and the juice from the mixture pressed out and strained with the fibers of *Cyperus laevigata*. A tablespoonful of the liquid thus obtained constitutes one dose and is taken three times a day—morning, noon, and evening, and as long as the supply lasts. When the supply is exhausted, another may be secured in the same manner. Five preparations of like amount may be made without causing any injury to the patient.

Again: For those affected with severe case of asthma which produces foul breath, the following mixture is recommended: Four pieces of the "kukui" bark the size of the palm of the hand; a like amount of the *Jambosa malecensis* and "koa" bark; a hatful of the stems and buds of the

Peperomia spp.; a similar amount of the stems and buds of the *Campylotheca;* two handsful of the "kohekohe" (small reeds that grow in bunches in taro patches); four fully matured *Morinda citrifolia* fruits; the bark of four *Waltheria americana* roots; a similar amount of the bark of the "popolo" roots; four segments of the white sugar-cane; four half-ripe *Morinda citrifolia* fruits. Have all these materials thoroughly pounded together and the juice from the mixture separated from the waste. This is strained with the fibers of the *Cyperus laevigata* and cooked with four red-hot stones. After the cooked liquid is cooled to the right temperature, the patient, lying down on his stomach with a cushion supporting his abdomen, drinks the whole of it. This is repeated morning and evening for five successive days. A fresh supply is needed for each dose. The *Campylotheca* tea should be taken regularly and, at the end, a good dose of a laxative. Sour poi and salty foods must be avoided.

Again: For scrofulous sores, bad cases of ulcer and other bad sores where the flesh seems to rot away, the following mixture is recommended: Take the meat of eight "kukui" nuts and have it baked in "ki" leaves until thoroughly cooked. This is pounded or finely ground and then set to one side. About a tablespoonful of the breadfruit milk is then secured and mixed with the prepared "kukui" meat. In the meantime about a spoonful of the finely ground *Cyperus laevigata* fibers and a like amount of the "lama" powder are being thoroughly mixed. The two mixtures are then put together and thoroughly stirred and applied by spreading it over the sore or sores. This is done morning and evening and as long as necessary.

Before the treatment, however, the sore should be washed with the tea of the *Bobea* spp. bark thoroughly cooked with about a gallon of water and with four red hot stones. The bark should be pounded before boiling it in order to get its strength.

Again: For swollen womb, the "kukui" shell is very helpful. A sufficient quantity of the shell is secured and put over live charcoals. A gourd, with narrow neck and with the inside partly scooped and cleaned is secured. The burning "kukui" shells are then thrown into it. As the smoke rises out of the opening at top of the neck, the patient, sitting on her heels with her legs spread far apart, allows as much of the "kukui" and gourd smoke or fume to enter her vagina. This produces the warmth and the effect which is beneficial to the womb. The treatment should be administered twice a day and for five successive days. The *Campylotheca* tea should be taken regularly by the patient.

And, again: For the purpose of building up the body after the system its free from its injurious poisons, etc., the following mixture is most effective: Take the meat of eight thoroughly baked "kukui" nuts and have them thoroughly ground. Bake about twelve very young taro leaves; mash about four or six very young shoots of the "kikawaioa" (no scientific name given) and then have all these materials mixed while the cooked "kukui" and the young taro leaves are still warm. This done, the patient, lying on his left side with a blanket supporting, eats the mixture thus prepared with potato poi mixed with the *Campylotheca* tea. This is done twice a day for five successive days. The *Campylotheca* tea should be used as a regular drink. Salty foods should be avoided. Together with the regular food, the papaia and banana should be eaten.

The oil of the "kukui" nut makes a very strong laxative. In case of using it, and if it works too freely, its action can be stopped by eating a couple of lumps of Hawaiian starch together with poi.

Another use of the "kukui" nut (when dried) is for lighting. The nuts are dried and strung together with the wire-like ribs of the cocoanut leaf and burnt like candles.

120. KUPALII or KUPAOA or AWA-LAU-A-KANE. (*Peperomia* sp.)

This plant grows on the side of cliffs and near the beach, and it is used as a remedy for the cure of asthma. The preparation is as follows: Take eight buds of the plant; two pieces of the mountain apple bark; the bark of eight *Waltheria americana* roots; a like amount of the "popolo" roots; the bark of eight *Sida* roots; a handful of the *Peperomia* spp. stems; four fully matured *Morinda citrifolia* fruits; one whole and partly dried cocoanut; four segments of the white sugar-cane. Have all these materials thoroughly pounded together and the juice pressed out and strained with the fibers of the *Cyperus laevigata*. Then put into the liquid about two good-sized red-hot stones with which to cook it. This done, the patient takes a drink of the liquid two times a day and for five successive days. Salty foods should be avoided by the patient. The cooked young taro leaves, fresh fish and the meat of the *Aleurites moluccana* nuts are good articles of food for the patient. The spring water should be regularly used instead of the other kind of water.

121. LAUKAHI or KUHEKILI. (No scientific name given.)

This plant does not grow very high. Its leaves are round and its small flowers come out in long clusters. It grows nearly everywhere in these islands. Its use as a remedy is for giving strength to those who are physically weak, especially the children. The application is as follows: For a child ten days old, one leaf is baked in the *Cordyline terminalis* leaves and then chewed by the mother and fed to the child. For one from twenty to forty days, a leaf and a half is taken and prepared in the same manner. For one from fifty days to three months, two whole leaves are given with the same manner of preparation; and for one from four to six months old, three leaves are given; while to one from seven months to one year old, four leaves are given. For a child above this age, it is better to give the *Peperomia* spp. preparation for the general debility of the body.

Another way of treating a child of ten days to six months old is by having the mother eat four leaves at a time with a piece of dried cocoanut. This she does morning and evening. The effect of the remedy will get to the child through the mother's milk and will be seen in the regularity with which the child's bowels move each day. The same effect will also be experienced by the mother. Should the bowels of the child move too freely, a check can be effected by the mother by discontinuing the use of the remedy.

For adults, four or more leaves (both green and dried) may be eaten at a time for softening the contents of the alimentary canal and for promoting regularity in the movement of the bowels. This remedy is about the easiest of all remedies to secure and to apply.

Another use of the leaves of this plant is the bringing to a head of a blind boil. For a large one, take two leaves and rub them together with some salt until they are softened. These are then put over the boil, covering the entire lump. A ring, made up of cloth wound around a core in the form of a ring, is put on and around the eye from which the pus might burst forth, and this is covered with a piece of cloth to keep it in place. This application is repeated every morning until the boil bursts open and the core removed. In the meantime it is well for the patient to take the *Impomea dissecta* to clean out the bowels.

122. LAUKAHI-LAUNUI. (No scientific name given.)

This plant is very much like the *Asplenium nidus*, only it is much smaller. It grows on trees. Its medicinal value and the way it is applied are very much the same as the *Asplenium nidus*.

123. LEPO-LOI or MAKUU. (No scientific name given.)

This is the black mud that is found in taro patches of long cultivation. This lies at the bottom of the soft mud over which the water stands. Together with the "waikoloa" or the small reeds that grow in taro patches, this mud makes a very good remedy for bad sores or openings at the bottom of the feet or under the armpit or about the chest. The sores are washed with the tea of the *Cassia occidentalis* and then left to dry. Half of a handful of the "waikoloa" reeds are then secured and thoroughly pounded into a sort of a paste. This is rubbed into the sores and covered with the mud. A piece of cloth is then wrapped around to keep the medicine in place. This is done in the morning and repeated in the evening, the application being continued for five successive days. During the treatment, the patient should keep his system clean and should take a good dose of laxative on the fourth day. Spring water only should be taken into the system.

Again: This mud is very helpful in the case of rupture. The following preparation is recommended: Take a handful of the "ki" shoots and a like amount of the "waikoloa" reeds. These are thoroughly pounded and put into a container. A handful of the mud is secured. The affected testicle is then lifted to allow the intestines to set back to their original place. The mixture of the "ki" shoots and the "waikoloa" reeds is placed under the testicle with two small pebbles supporting and closing into the rupture. The mud then is appled over the pebbles and this is supported by a piece of cloth after a leaf of the *Morinda citrifolia* is laid over it. If the *Morinda citrifolia* leaf cannot be secured, use a round cabbage leaf. This treatment is repeated every morning for five successive days. Laxative should be taken by the patient every two days. For drinking, the spring water should be used, also the *Campylotheca* tea. Articles of food are the same as those recommended for the other treatments.

124. LIMU-EKAHA. (No scientific name given.)

This moss grows on rotted trees. It is flat like a ribbon and is greenish in color. The moss is bitter both in green and dry state. As a remedy, it is good for diseased growth of the skin. The following is the preparation: Take about a tablespoonful of the powder of the moss; a like amount of the powdered "lama" wood; and a tablespoonful of the breadfruit milk. These are thoroughly mixed and, after the growth or diseased portion of the skin is washed with the tea of the *Cassia occidentalis*, the mixture is rubbed into the affected part. The treatment is applied morning and evening for five successive days.

Another mixture recommended is that of about a tablespoonful of the powdered moss and a like amount of the copper dust. This is applied in the same way as the other mixture.

Laxative should be taken every three days and the articles of food for the patient are the same as those recommended for the other treatments.

125. LIMU OPULEPULE. (No scientific name given.)

This moss has spots from which it derives its name. It grows in swampy ground and on rocks. It is not bitter. Its medicinal value and use are the same as the former moss, "limu ekaha."

126. LIMU-KALAWAI. (No scientific name given.)

This water weed, a good article of food, grows in fish-ponds almost anywhere around these islands. It is used as a remedy for the relief of the burning effect which frequently occurs about the chest. The preparation is as follows: Take the weed and chop it to an amount equal to about a quart. Add to this eight very young "kikawaiaoa" stems and shoots and four thoroughly baked *Aleurites moluccana* nut meat. Have these materials thoroughly pounded together and put into a container. Add to the mixture eight baked young taro leaves and have the whole thing well mixed. The patient then lies down on his stomach with a cushion supporting his chest and eats the mixture either with fresh poi or baked sweet potato. Spring water should be taken regularly and a laxative at the end of the treatment, which is taken twice a day for five consecutive days.

127. LIMU-KALA-KAI. (No scientific name.)

This sea-weed is rough in appearance. Its pea-like seeds come in clusters. It is a good article of food. This, and the "lipoa" or fragrant sea weed, chewed together with baked taro by the mother and fed to the child forty days old, makes a good remedy for bodily weakness. This treatment is given twice a day and is continued until the child is about six months old.

128. LIMU MAKOLEMAKAOPII or KALEMAKAPII.
(No scientific name given.)

This water weed is of a very dark green color and grows near or about springs. The flowers are white and sometimes yellow. The value of this weed as a medicine is like the above. The preparation is as follows: Take about a quartful of the weed; twelve very young shoots of the *Cyperus laevigata;* about a tablespoonful of the coral powder and a like amount of the tortoise shell powder (very fine scrapings of the shell). Have all these materials carefully wrapped in "ki" leaves and baked. When the mixture is cooked, make a small opening in the side of the bundle and, as the steam issues forth, direct it to the eyes of the patient. This done, squeeze the juice of the cooked mixture out and put it in a container from which it is taken by the patient. This is followed by eating baked sweet potato. For adults, the mixture may be boiled and the tea from it taken as in the case of the *Campylotheca* tea. For convenience, it is well to have these materials collected, dried and put away ready for use at any time.

129. LIMU-KELE. (No scientific name given.)

This is a black and rather tough water weed which grows in taro patches and in running streams. It is almost tasteless. This weed is used for young women whose menstruation has just begun. The following is the preparation: Take about a quartful of the weed and have it chopped and dried. This, then, is ground into powder and mixed with about a teaspoonful of the "limu-makolemakaopii" powder and about two pints of the clay and sufficient amount of water. The patient then drinks the whole of the mixture and this is followed by eating warm baked sweet potato. This dose is taken twice a day for five consecutive days. Laxative should be taken at the end of five days; and should the treatment be continued for some time after the first five days are ended (a practice which is often carried out in order to prevent occurrence of sharp severe pains when menstruation takes place), care of the body and of the food should be particularly observed. The *campylotheca* tea should be regularly taken and all salty foods with moderation. Baked taro, sweet potato and young taro leaves are good articles of food.

130. LIMU-LIPOA-KUAHIWI. (No scientific name given.)

This is mountain weed and it is somewhat similar to the fragrant sea weed "lipoa" in general appearance. Its leaves are green and shiny. Its taste is somewhat salty and puckery. This weed is largely used for those afflicted with sores in the mouth, especially the children. It is also used for children having weakness of the body.

The following is the preparation: Take about a quartful of the weed and a similar amount of the "lipoa" or fragrant sea-weed and have these thoroughly dried out in the sun. In the meantime, a tablespoonful of the "lama" wood powder and a like amount of the *Cyperus laevigata* powder are secured; also the juice of four *Aleurites moluccana* nuts and a tablespoonful of the milk of the breadfruit. Have all these materials thoroughly mixed into a paste and then spread over the sores of the lips or mouth of the patient. This treatment is given morning and evening and is continued until the sores are healed.

131. LIMU-LIPOA-KAI. (No scientific name given.)

This sea-weed grows in shallow water along the beach, usually on coral where the breakers go over. It is fragrant and is eaten as food. Its medicinal value and application are like the above weed, the "limu-lipoa-kuahiwi."

132. LIMU-ELEELE-KAI. (No scientific name given.)

This is water weed (although frequently found growing at mouths of streams or rivers where fresh and salt water meet) and it is largely used as food. Its color is deep green and is very slippery. It is found at Moanalua and Kalia and is frequently sold at the fishmarket as food. Mixed with other medicines, it becomes very effective for the removal of white blotches on the skin.

The following is the preparation: Take a quartful of the weed; the bark of eight *Waltheria americana* roots; the bark of eight "popolo" roots; two pieces of the mountain apple bark; two segments of the white sugar-cane and a quartful of water. The different pieces of bark and the sugar cane segments are then thoroughly pounded together and then mixed with the water and the weed. These are then cooked with six red-hot stones; and, after being cooked, the liquid from the mixture is separated and strained with the fine fibers of the *Cyperus laevigata*. The patient takes a mouthful of this liquid for a single dose. This is repeated twice a day for five consecutive days. Salty foods must be avoided. Laxative should be taken after the treatments are over and the *Campylotheca* tea should regularly be used.

133. LIMU-LIPALA-WAI. (No scientific name given.)

This water weed is somewhat similar to the former, differing only in the color at the tip, which is yellowish. Like the former, this also is used as food. The use of the weed as a medicine is for the removal of the congestion about the chest. It is prepared as follows: Take about a quartful of the weed and, after removing all the water from it, put it together with twelve young taro leaves. These are wrapped in "ki" leaves and baked over the charcoal fire. At the same time, the slimy substance of the very young fern leaves or shoots is being secured and made ready in a wooden dish. When the weed and young taro leaves are cooked, they are mixed with this slimy substance and a little salt and eaten by the patient with poi or baked sweet potato. This is repeated twice a day for five days in succession. The treatment, however, could be continued after this time. At the end of the fifth day, the *Impomea dissecta* should be taken as a laxative.

134. LIMU-LI-PALAHALAHA. (No scientific name given.)

This water weed grows most abundantly in rivers. It is deep green in color and quite puffed in the appearance of its size,—a factor which distinguishes it from the other woods of similar make-up. It is used as food and is taken with warm pork or beef stew. By mixing it with the young taro leaves and then baked, it becomes very helpful for stomach ache. It is taken two times a day and for five successive days. After this, the *Impomea dissecta* is taken for washing the bowels.

135. LIMU-LI-PUU-PUU. (No scientific name given.)

This sea-weed grows on nearly all the reefs along the shores of these islands. It has seeds that are lumpy in appearance and they bear great similarity to the seeds of the *Psilotum triquetrum*. In looks, it is rough, but it is a very good article of food. Its odor is somewhat fragrant. This weed is used for the relief of those affected with bodily weakness, especially the children. The following is the preparation for the children:

The mother takes the weed and chews it with baked sweet potato to fill about a tablespoon, and then the mixture is fed to the child twice a day for five successive days. This dose is suitable for any child from sixty days to one year old.

When the child discharges from his system small lumps together with the chewed weed and potato, then it is time for some laxative to be given to him for internal cleaning. This the mother does by taking the laxative herself and the child from her through her breast. But, should the child's physical condition allow, he may take the laxative directly.

136. LIMU LI-PAAKAI. (No scientific name given.)

This sea-weed grows on coral and rocks at the water's edge, usually just where the waves break. The name applies to the state when it is not detached from the rocks When it is, it takes the name "limukohu" (or the weed that has stain) It is a very good article of food. It is bitter in taste but, if allowed to be in fresh water over night, it loses its bitterness. It is frequently eaten with raw fish such as "oio" or "awa-aua."

The use of this weed as a remedy is for the purpose of healing a sprain, relieving stomach ache, pain about the wrist and knee and back ache. The following is the preparation: Take about a quart of the weed; twelve green and twelve ripe leaves of the *Morinda citrifolia* and have these materials thoroughly pounded together. The paste-like mixture is then applied directly by spreading it over the injured part and then wrapping a bandage around to keep the remedy in place. Another way of applying is by putting the mixture in a piece of cloth and then rubbing the injured part with it three times a day for five successive days. Laxative should be taken by the patient every three days until complete relief is experienced.

137. LIMU-LI-PEHU. (No scientific name given.)

This sea weed may be found on reefs in shallow water along the shores of these islands. The growth is rugged and rough and is somewhat scattered. As a remedy, it is effective for the cure of white blotches on the skin or for rash. It is largely used by those who live along the shore. The following is the preparation: Take a quart of the weed; the bark of eight *Cassia occidentalis* roots; four "kupukupu" plants; four "haukeuke" or sea-egg shells; two spoonsful of ashes; four spoonsful of Hawaiian salt and a half of a tablespoonful of red sugar-cane juice. Have all these materials thoroughly pounded together and put in a piece of cloth. The remedy is then rubbed over the afflicted part morning, noon and evening until cured. A single preparation is sufficient for one day's application.

138. LIMU-LUAU. (No scientific name given.)

This sea-weed grows in very deep water. It derives its name from the fact that, in general appearance, it resembles the nature of baked or cooked young taro leaves. The only opportunity for securing it is when the ocean is rough. It is then detached from the rocks and taken to the shore by the current. As a remedy, it is helpful for trouble about the chest. It may be prepared as follows: A quart of the weed; four very young taro leaves and a handful of the young potato leaves. Scrape into the mixture some fully matured cocoanut meat and then have the whole thing wrapped in "ki" leaves and baked. After being cooked, the patient eats the mixture with baked taro morning and evening for five successive days. Laxative should be taken at the end of the treatment. Spring water should be used during the entire treatment.

139. LIMU-MANAUEA. (No scientific name given.)

This sea weed grows on reef along the shore, in shallow water. It is pinkish in color and somewhat rugged and scattered in appearance. It is usually cooked with stewed beef or with squid. As a remedy, it is largely employed for the cure of miscarriage. The following is the preparation: Take a quartful of the weed; eight very young taro leaves; about a half of a hatful of the very young potato leaves and a similar amount of the "pakapakai." Have these materials cooked and put into a container with sufficient amount of water for broth. The entire content is then seasoned with a little salt and eaten with potato by the patient. This is done two times a day and for five successive days. On the sixth day, the *Impomea dissecta* is taken for a laxative. During the treatment, spring water should be used. Poi may be taken if it is not sour.

140. LIMU-PAHAPAHA-KAI. (No scientific name given.)

This sea weed, having the appearance of thin curled paper and green in color, grows most abundantly at the edge of the water along the shores of these islands. It is used as food. Its use as a remedy is for the relief of those affected with asthma, especially those having very severe cases. This is the preparation and treatment:

Take a quart of the weed; sixteen leaves of the *Desmodium uncinatum;* and a quartful of the buds and flowers of the *Waltheria americana*. Have these materials thoroughly dried out in the sun and then crushed or ground into a sort of very coarse powder to be used in a pipe. The patient then smokes this powdered mixture from four to five times a day for five successive days. After this period, he takes the finely ground raw potato with warm water in order to stimulate vomiting. This is done in order to remove the phlegm from the stomach and lungs. A continuation of the treatment after this is not prohibited. Laxative should be used after the treatment and the tea from the mixture of equal parts of the *Campylotheca* and the *Psilotum triquetrum* leaves in a quart of boiling water should be used regularly.

141. LIMU-PAHAPAHA-WAI. (No scientific name given.)

This weed resembles the preceding in every way, the only difference being that the former grows in salt water while this grows in fresh water. The medicinal value and use of the two are alike.

142. LIMU-HUNA. (No scientific name given.)

This sea weed is very fine in appearance and grows in hollows in coral reefs. The Hawaiians use it as food and is cooked together with squid. As a remedy, it is used for the cure of disorder in the alimentary canal. To prepare it.

Take a quartful of the weed; a small squid; forty medium-sized abalone; and a quart of water. Have these things boiled and, after being cooked and cooled to the right temperature, the patient then lies down on his stomach with a cushion supporting his abdomen, and drinks the broth and eats the squid and abalone with either poi or sweet potato, and baked young taro leaves or luau. The *Campylotheca* tea should be taken as a regular drink. The following day laxative should be taken to clean the bowels. Three days after the first dose another should be taken and so on until five are taken.

143. LOULU-LELO. (No scientific name given.)

This tree grows to a tremendous size and resembles the "kauwila" in general appearance. The trunk and leaves are of very rich brown color. The leaves are like those of the "kamani" and so are the seeds. It grows anywhere among the mountains of these islands. The bud and the meat of the seed are used for the general weakness of the body. It is prepared thus:

For a child ten days old, have the mother chew two buds, a piece of dried cocoanut meat and the meat of two seeds and feed the juice of the mixture to the child. This is followed by feeding with the mother's milk. For a child from thirty to sixty days old, the juice of four buds and a like amount of the meat of the seeds and a piece of dried cocoanut is given. For a child from six months to one year old, the following is prepared and given:

Take eight buds and a like amount of the meat of the seeds and a piece of dried cocoanut. Add to these materials, one segment of the white sugar-cane; a piece of the bark of the mountain apple; a handful of the *Peperomia* spp.; one half-ripe and one fully matured *Morinda citrifolia* fruit. Have these materials thoroughly pounded together and the juice from the mixture pressed out and strained with the fibers of the *Cyperus laevigata*. A tablespoonful of this liquid is taken by the patient three times a day and as long as necessary. When the supply is consumed, another may be prepared in the same way.

144. LEKO-ELEELE. (No scientific name given, but commonly known as watercress.)

The watercress is found in patches, streams and ditches. It is used as food and is especially good when boiled with pork. As a remedy, it is helpful for severe cases of asthma. It is prepared as follows: Four hatsful of the watercress; one dried cocoanut; the bark of four *Waltheria americana* roots; a like amount of each of the "puakala," "popolo" and mountain apple bark and one and a half segments of the white sugar cane, are all put together and thoroughly pounded. The juice from the mixture is then pressed out and strained with the fibers of the *Cyperus laevigata*. In the meantime, a spoonful of the clay powder is being secured and this is put into the juice and mixed. The whole thing is then boiled with a red-hot stone thrown into it. After being cooked and cooled to the right temperature, the patient drinks the whole of it. In the evening of the same day, another dose is prepared and taken. This is repeated for five successive days. The *Campylotheca* tea should be used regularly and, at the end of the treatment, the *Impomea dissecta* is taken as a laxative. During the treatment, salty foods should be avoided, also the fish having dark flesh. Fresh poi and broiled fresh fish can be taken.

145. LEKO-KEOKEO. (White watercress.) (No scientific name given.)

This watercress resembles the former in every way except the color and taste,—the former being dark and bitter while the latter is light and not so bitter. Like the former, it is an article of food. As a remedy, it is good for cold in the head and for dry throat. Take about twenty young branches and eat all of them at the same time with a piece of dried cocoanut. This is repeated three or four times a day and as long as necessary. For a cold of long duration it is necessary to take two tablespoonsful of salt water every three days. The *Campylotheca* tea should be taken regularly and when it is warm. Baked taro or sweet potato and baked young taro leaves and "kukui" nut meat are good articles of food to take during the treatment. Salty foods should be avoided. The bowels should move regularly.

146. LIMU-ONOHI-AWA. (No scientific name given.)

This is black moss which grows around stones and boulders in streams and rivers; also in fish ponds. It is shiny and somewhat puffed up while in water, thus presenting a size much larger than what it really is. Like the above-mentioned weeds, this moss is used for food. As a remedy this moss is good for the cure of bad sores, ulcers and ragged cuts. It is prepared as follows:

Take a quartful of the moss; a like amount of the *Panicum pruricus*; some tobacco leaves and some "lama" wood. Have all these materials thoroughly dried and, with the exception of the "lama" wood, which is scraped until a tablespoonful of its dust is secured, have them burnt separately and get from each a tablespoonful of the ashes. This done, the ashes are thrown together and mixed with the "lama" wood dust and the milk of two papaia fruits. The mixture is then applied to the sore by spreading it. The *Impomea dissecta* is taken every four days for cleaning the system.

147. LUMAHA'I. (No scientific name given.)

This tree grows most abundantly on Kauai. The wood is very hard. The bark is light and very smooth. The bud and the fruit of this tree are very useful for the cure of internal disorders. The following is the preparation:

Take four buds and four fruits and eat them with a piece of fully matured cocoanut. This is followed by eating the baked young taro leaves with the baked sweet potato. This constitutes one dose and is repeated twice a day and for five successive days. Should the remedy become too laxative, the patient may rest for a while and, should the bowels move too freely, four lumps of Hawaiian starch may be eaten with poi and this will stop the loose action of the remedy. A regular opening medicine may be taken after this to thoroughly rid the system of any weakening effect from the medicine. The *Campylotheca* tea should be taken regularly.

For purifying the blood, the bark, especially that portion closest the soil or the bark of the roots, is very effective when mixed with the other remedies. This is the preparation:

Take four pieces of the bark the size of the palm of the hand; a like amount of the *Bobea* spp. bark; eight *Curcuma louza* bulbs; the meat of the *Cibatium vhamissoi kaulf.* about sixteen inches long; the "ti" root of the same size; a piece of the *Impomea dissecta;* a half-ripe *Morinda citrifolia* fruit; two segments of the red sugar-cane; about a quartful of the leaves and flowers of the *Campylotheca;* a handful of the *Psilotum triquetrum* and two pieces of the "koa" bark. Have all these materials thoroughly pounded together and put into a container of about two and a half quarts of water. The whole thing then is cooked with twelve red-hot stones,—the container being covered steam tight after the stones are put in. After being cooked and cooled, the fibers and solid materials are removed and the remaining liquid strained with the fibers of the *Cyperus laevigata* and put into another container which could be tightly covered. The patient then takes a mouthful of this liquid three times a day. At the end of the fourth day, he should take some opening medicine. Salty foods should be avoided, also fish having dark flesh. The young taro leaves, the *Aleurites* nuts, banana, potato and poi with baked fish are good articles of food.

148. MAUNALOA. (No scientific name given.)

This plant grows like a vine and resembles the growth of the *Impomea dissecta.* The leaves are round and can be found anywhere. The leaves and roots of the plant are effective for deep cuts. The following is the preparation: Take a quartful of the leaves; eight roots; about a pint of Hawaiian salt and have all these materials thoroughly pounded together and wrapped with the fibers of the cocoanut. The juice then is squeezed out and allowed to flow into the cut. This is done morning and evening for five successive days. But should the the wound heal before this time further application of the remedy will not be necessary. At the end, however, laxative should be taken by the patient. After the system is cleansed a blood-purifying remedy must be taken. The patient must not eat very salty foods. The *Campylotheca* tea should be taken regularly.

The seed of this plant is very effective for blood purifying and for destroying worms. This is the preparation: Two to four seeds may be taken and eaten three to four times a day. Should they be too laxative, the patient may rest for a while. Whatever the case may be, the eating of the seeds is very beneficial to the general health of the patient.

The leaves of this plant are good for the cure of skin eruptions and skin diseases. The patient may eat four green leaves three to four times a day. Another way of applying is by bathing. Forty large leaves are taken; a similar amount of the *Dodonaea ciscosa* leaves; forty leaves of the *Tephrosia piscatoria;* four *Cassia occidentalis* plants. Have these materials thoroughly pounded together and put into a container of water into which eight red-hot stones are submerged. After the content is cooked and cooled, the fibers may be removed and the liquid emptied into another container. The patient then bathes his body with this liquid twice a day for five successive days. The *Campylotheca* tea may be taken as a regular drink and, at the end, a good dose of a laxative.

149. MAIA—MAIA-LELE. (*Musa sapientum*, many varieties)

This banana is low in height and it derives its name from the fact that its flowers fall off very early. The juice from the bud or young flower is good for the removal of the weakness of the body arising from stomach disorder, thus producing white coating over the tongue. The bud may be secured and the tip cut off. The juice which comes from the cut is taken and rubbed on the tongue and the entire interior of the mouth. This is done three times a day and, during the treatment, the tongue may be gently scraped in order to remove the white covering hardened by the medicine. Laxative must be taken every three days. When the tongue shows a clean reddish appearance, it is indicative that the system has rid itself of the cause of the ailment. The treatment, therefore, may be discontinued.

150. MAIA-MAOLI. (No scientific name given.)

This banana grows most abundantly in Kona, Hawaii. The tree grows to considerable height and quite large in size. The banana itself is large and very delicious. It is good for sickly people. As a remedy, it is specially useful for the relief of cramps in the stomach, etc. The following is the preparation: Take the bud and have the upper half cut off and then add to it these materials: The ink sack of the dried squid; a lump of red clay; and a quartful of the buds and green leaves of the "popolo," also a taro leaf. Have these things thoroughly but separately pounded and then mixed. The juice then is squeezed out and strained with the fibers of the *Cyperus laevigata*. This constitutes one dose and is taken by the patient just as soon as cleaned. This is repeated twice a day and for five successive days. After the treatment, the *Impomea dissecta* is taken for a laxative. The *Campylotheca* tea, mixed with that of the *Psilotum triquetrum*, should be taken regularly.

151. MAIA-IHOLENA. (No scientific name given.)

This banana is yellowish in color and it derives its name from this fact. It grows anywhere among the mountains of these islands and it is a cherished food of the ancient native birds of Hawaii nei. The tree is not very high and the leaves are somewhat yellowish; also the trunk. Its value as a remedy is very much the same as the "maia-lele." In this case, however, both the bud and the portion of the trunk closest the ground are used for the cure of disorders arising from the stomach and the alimentary canal. This portion of the banana is cut and the surface where the knife has gone through is turned up in order to hold the juice. The juice of two green *Aleurites moluccana* nuts then is mixed with that of the banana and the mixture is immediately applied by rubbing the child's tongue or lips or between the fingers or toes or wherever the internal disorder has broken out.

152. MAIA-KOAE. (No scientific name given.)

The trunk of this banana is high and its leaves and trunk are lined with white stripes. The fruit bears the same characteristic. The fully matured banana is good, when mixed with other remedies, for stubborn case of constipation. The following is the mixture:

Take the meat of four fully matured bananas and scape them into a container; the meat of one taro ("lauloa") and treat it in the same manner; the meat of two *Aleurites moluccana* nuts; the slimy substance of the *Hibiscus tiliaceus* from two pieces of the bark; two clusters of the *Aleurites moluccana* flowers and a pint of spring water. The solid matter, after being crushed thoroughly, is mixed with the water. In the meantime, the bark of the mountain apple is being pounded with one segment of the white sugar-cane. This mixture is put together with the rest and stirred and then a red-hot stone is put in to cook the entire content. This done, the fibers are removed and the liquid cleaned and strained with fresh fibers of the *Cyperus laevigata*. The patient then takes the entire dose in the morning. When the bowels begin to move, then the patient is given eight thoroughly baked *Impomea dissecta* buds and warm dose of the *Campylotheca* tea.

153. MAI'A-HA-A. (No scientific name given.)

This banana is not very high and grows very much like the "iholena" and "lele." The trunk is rather dark. The bud or the very young cluster as it begins to come forth, from the tree, and the young tree or the offspring from the parent stock, are very helpful for internal disorders causing general debility of the body. The following is the preparation:

Take the bud and cut it about two inches from the biggest end. Do the same with the young banana tree. As the juice from both comes out, it is collected into a container and mixed with the juice of four young *Aleurites moluccana* nuts and two half-ripe papaia fruits. The mixture then is rubbed on the tongue and roof of the mouth of the afflicted child or person. Before applying, however, it is well to rid the tongue of the white coating which usually covers its surface when such ailment takes place.

154. MAIA ELEELE. (No scientific name given.)

This banana has dark color and this fact makes it different from other bananas. The fibers from the covering of the trunk is frequently made into hats. Its value as a remedy and the way it is applied are very much like those described above. The leaves, however, are usually burnt and the ashes sprinkled on the poi and eaten by the patient. This is followed by a drink of water.

153. MAIA KAHIKI. (No scientific name given.)

This banana is quite large in size and the covering of the trunk is somewhat reddish. As a remedy, it is of very small value. The "kahunas" or the medicine men of old used this banana in their practices as a part of their rituals.

154. MAIA-MANAI-ULA. (No scientific name given.)

This banana is quite large in size and the fruit is very much like the "popoulu" banana. The color is pink. The leaves are marked with white streaks at the center and the inside of the fruit is whitish. This kind of banana is fast becoming scarce.

The half-ripe or fully matured banana is used for the cure of different kinds of asthma. The preparation and application are as follows:

Take four fully matured bananas and have the inside or the meat scraped into a container; take one sweet potato the size of the fist and have this scraped and mixed with the banana; then take four half-ripe *Morinda citrifolia* fruits; two segments of the white or red sugar-cane and one fully matured cocoanut and have these thoroughly pounded together and the juice therefrom pressed out and strained with the fibers of the *Cyperus laevigata*. In the meantime a lump of red clay the size of the *Aleurites* nut is being mixed with a sufficient amount of water. All these materials are then thoroughly mixed and again strained with the fibers of the *Cyperus laevigata*. The liquid from this entire mixture constitutes one dose and is taken at one time. The patient should take two doses a day—morning and evening, for five successive days. The *Impomea dissecta* should be taken for a laxative after the last dose is taken.

155. MAIA-POPOULU. (No scientific name given.)

This banana resembles the "maoli" in general appearance. Its fruit is shorter and quite large in size. The meat is very much like that of the breadfruit in color. As a remedy, its value, use and application are similar to those of the "maoli." But the root of the young shoot of this banana, when mixed with other remedies, becomes very effective for the cure of asthma or troubles about the chest. The following is the preparation:

Take one young shoot; the bark of eight roots of the *Waltheria americana;* the bark of eight "puakala" roots; two pieces of the bark of the mountain apple the size of the palm of the hand; the same amount of the *Aleurites moluccana* bark; two handsful of the small taro patch reeds known as the "kohekohe"; about a quart of the flowers, buds and leaves of the "popolo" and three segments of the white sugar-cane. Have all these materials thoroughly pounded together and the juice therefrom strained with the fibers of the *Cyperus laevigata*. This done, put into the liquid about two red-hot stones to cook it. After cooking, the liquid is allowed to cool and is taken by the patient at night for five successive nights.

156. MAIA-POPOULU-LAHI. (No scientific name given.)

This banana is like the preceding in every way except its leaves, and the outside of the fruit is very thin. As a remedy it is good for the destruction of worms that cause itch about the rectum. This is the preparation:

Take four young fruits; two *Impomea dissecta* vines about the size of the thumb and about eight inches long; one sweet potato about the size of the fist with the outside removed; two fully matured fruits of the *Morinda citrifolia;* a piece of the *Hibiscus tiliaceus* bark the size of the palm of the hand; two segments of the white sugar-cane; a small lump of the red clay; a piece of the mountain apple bark. Have all these materials thoroughly pounded together and put into a container. Have the very coarse materials removed and the remainder put into the fibers of the *Cyperus laevigata* and the liquid therefrom pressed out and strained. This constitutes one dose and is taken in the morning. Another is taken at night and is repeated for five successive days. Much spring water should be taken by the patient. At the proper time, or, when constipated, laxative should be taken. There are no food restrictions.

157. MAIA-PUAPUA-NUI. (No scientific name given.)

This banana looks very much like the "lele" banana and is not so very large in size. The fruit is large and roundish in shape. The flowers are large and they remain on the fruit to maturity, hence the name. The young cluster, as it emerges from the trunk and takes on the shape of a bud, is good for the cure of the general weakness of the body. It removes from the system the impurities which cause the run-down condition of the body. The following is the preparation: Take the bud and cut it near the tip. Take out from the two surfaces all the juice that comes from them to the extent of two tablespoonsful. This then is mixed with a small lump of red clay and some coral powder, also some drops from two young *Aleurites moluccana* nuts. This mixture constitutes one dose and is rubbed into the tongue of the patient, also on the temple, on the fore part of the head and on the navel.

158. MAIA-PALAHOLO-PALAKAHUKI. (No scientific name given.)

This is a banana tree the fruit of which is taken off and is left standing until it begins to rot. This trunk is good for the cure of the burning effect in the chest or about the stomach. It is also used for those affected with excessive perspiration. The following is the preparation:

Take about a quart of the softened portion of the trunk and mix it with a like amount of the slimy substance of the *Hibiscus tiliaceus*. Add to these the dark clay to the amount of two teaspoonsful; a like amount of the red clay; the juice of one segment of the white sugar-cane and about four very young shoots of the eating fern. The whole thing then is put into the fibers of the *Cyperus laevigata* and strained. The resulting liquid is divided into two equal parts, one to be taken by the patient in the morning and the other in the evening, for five successive days. After the last dose is taken, usually the day after, laxative is taken to clean the bowels. The *Campylotheca* tea should be taken regularly.

159. MAIA—PILALI and LAUHULU. (No scientific name given.)

The sweet juice from the banana flowers and the dried leaves are good remedies for different kinds of asthma when mixed with other remedies. The following is the preparation:

Take about four tablespoonsful of the sweet juice from the banana flowers and empty them into a pint of water, allowing the same to remain there overnight. Then take about a quartful of the young *Portulaca oleracea;* eight fully matured *Morinda citrifolia* fruits; two pieces of the mountain apple bark the size of the palm of the hand; four medium-sized clusters of the *Aleurites moluccana* flowers; the half of the meat of the fully matured cocoanut that is roasted until partly burnt; four roasted *Aleurites moluccana* nuts; two handsful of the *Peperomia* spp.; one *Curcuma louza* bulb; a lump of the red clay the size of a nut; four segments of the white sugar-cane. Have all these materials thoroughly pounded together and then mixed with the banana flower juice that is mixed with the water as above given. The juice from the entire mixture then is pressed out and strained with the fibers of the *Cyperus laevigata* and allowed to stand in a tightly corked bottle. In the meantime, the dried leaves of the banana and those of the "pili" are being separately burnt and a tablespoonful of the ashes of each being secured. These are mixed with the liquid.

The patient takes a mouthful of the preparation for a single dose and this is repeated three times a day until the entire amount is consumed. Food restrictions are the same as those connected with the remedies already given. In this case, however, much "iholena" and "lele" bananas should be eaten.

160. MAILE-KUAHIWI. (*Alyxia clivaeformis*)

There are different kinds of "maile," some having large leaves and some small, but their odor, their use by the Hawaiians as wreaths and their medicinal value are alike. The use of this vine in sweat bath is for the removal of the yellowish blotches on the skin. The following is the preparation:

Take two hatsful of the "maile"; a like amount of the kind having a strong and disagreeable odor; four *Cassia occidentalis* plants; and a hatful of the "kukaepipi" grass. These materials are then crushed by pounding them together and put into a container having about two or three quarts of water. Four red-hot stones are dropped into the mixture and as the water begins to boil, the patient, sitting in front of the container, covers himself with heavy blankets and allows the steam to go all over his body. As the perspiration flows from the body it is immediately removed with a towel and this is kept up until the sweating ceases. As the liquid cools, four more red-hot stones are put into it to keep up the steam. When the sweating ceases, the patient may bathe his body with the liquid.

In olden days, this treatment was employed wholly by the rulers of the land and not by the subjects. The name by which this form of treatment was known was "kili-kili-oe."

161. MAILE-KALUHEA. (*Coprosma* sp.)

This vine grows among cliffs and its odor is very disagreeable. As a remedy it is very good for ulcers and scrofulous sores. The tea from this vine is used as a wash. The following is the preparation: Take two hatsful of the vine and roots; four *Cassia occidentalis* plants; four pieces of the *Bobea* spp. bark and two of the *Acacia koa*. Have these materials thoroughly pounded together and put into a container having about two quarts of water. Then put into it four red-hot stones and have the container tightly covered. Allow the content to become thoroughly cooked. Additional stones may be added in order to bring this about. After being cooked, the liquid is strained with the fibers of the *Cyperus laevigata* and put into another container. The wound or sore is then washed with as much of the liquid as necessary. The patient should take the *Campylotheca* tea regularly and some laxative at the end of every four days. Salty foods should be avoided, also sour poi. Cooked fresh foods and bananas should be freely eaten. This liquid is good not only as a wash but for removing skin diseases.

162. MA-O. (*Abutilon incanum*)

This plant grows wild and its general appearance is something like the hibiscus. The leaves are quite large and the flowers are somewhat yellowish. The wood is very tough and the juice from it is very bitter. The flowers and the bark of the roots of this plant are used for the cure of gripping stomach ache. The following is the preparation:

Take twenty "ma-o" flowers; twenty hibiscus flowers, (using only the white of the base of the flowers); twenty "nohu" flowers; a like amount of the *Sida* flowers and a piece of cocoanut meat. These are partly dried and eaten by the patient. In the meantime the following preparation is being made ready: The bark of four "ma-o" roots; a like amount of the bark of the *Waltheria americana* roots, also of the "popolo" roots; a piece of the mountain apple bark; a half of a segment of the red sugar-cane; and a piece of the *Impomea dissecta* root. These are thoroughly pounded together with a piece of cocoanut and emptied into a container having about two pints of water and the liquid thus obtained strained with the fibers of the *Cyperus laevigata*. This liquid is then cooked with a red-hot stone thrown into it. As the flowers are eaten (twelve of each for a single dose) a mouthful of this liquid is taken. This constitutes the first dose. The second dose is made up of eight flowers of each kind chewed with a piece of cocoanut and, like the first, a mouthful of the liquid follows. In case of some left over of the liquid, this may be taken the next day. Laxative may be taken on the fourth day but, should internal disorder occur before that time, a dose of it should be taken immediately with the enema following. Salt water should be used for the injection. The patient may eat any article of food which his appetite requires.

163. MAUU LA-ILI. (No scientific name given.)

This form of grass is very scarce and may be found on Haleakala, Hualalai and Waialeale. The leaves resemble those of the onion. In olden days, the grass was in abundance at Kanaio, Maui. As a remedy, this grass is very effective for skin diseases. It draws the poison from the skin and removes whatever scales that have formed on it. The following is the preparation:

Take a hatful of the grass; a few grains of salt; a half of a segment of white sugar-cane and the bark of two roots of the *Cassia occidentalis*. Have these materials thoroughly pounded together and wrapped in the fine fibers of the cocoanut. The juice from the bulk is squeezed out and on the affected parts of the skin. This is rubbed into the skin. The treatment is repeated four or five times a day and at the end of two days the affected part or parts are washed with the tea of the *Bobea* spp. mixed with the "aiea." Salty foods should be avoided, also sour poi. Cooked fresh fish, baked young taro leaves, baked meat of the *Aleurites moluccana* nuts and the baked young "popolo" leaves are good articles of food to be consumed. The *Campylotheca* tea should be taken regularly and at the end of the fourth day the bowels should be cleaned with a good laxative.

164. MAKA-LOA. (No scientific name given.)

This reed grows in bunches to the height of about three feet. When dried, it makes good material for hat and mat weaving. The expensive Niihau mats are made of this material. This reed grows in swamps. As a remedy, it is good for the cure of difficulty in discharging urine. The following is the preparation:

Take a handful of the reed, removing the portion just above the roots; a piece of the "awa" root about the size of the fist; the white portion at the bottom of eight very young shoots of the "ti" or *Cordyline terminalis;* one bulb of the *Curcuma louza;* a lump of red clay about the size of the *Aleurites moluccana* nut and a like amount of the dark tough clay. Have all these materials thoroughly pounded together and the liquid therefrom strained with the fibers of the *Cyperus laevigata*. This constitutes one dose. The patient is given two doses a day—one in the morning and one in the evening—and these are continued for five consecutive days. Spring water should be taken in considerable amount, also the *Campylotheca* tea. Salty foods should be avoided. Taking the "iholena" and "lele" bananas for food is strongly recommended.

165. MAKI-A-WAHINE. (No scientific name given.)

This plant grows into a bush, thriving most favorably along hillsides and cliffs. Of late, however, this plant has become very scarce. Some people call it grass, the general appearance being that of the *Panicum pruricus*. As a remedy, the use of this plant is good for the cure of scaly skin or for skin disease. This is the preparation:

Take a quartful of the buds and leaves of the plant and a handful of the roots; the meat of eight *Aleurites moluccana* nuts; a handful of the "kupukupu hohono"; the bark of eight matured roots of the *Cassia occidentalis;* the milk of two fully matured papais; four mountain ginger bulbs; a like amount of the *Curcuma louza* bulbs; one matured *Morinda citrifolia* fruit and a sufficient amount of Hawaiian salt. Have these materials thoroughly pounded together and the juice therefrom strained with the fibers of the *Cyperus laevigata*. The juice is then applied as a wash for the affected parts of the body from three to six times a day. If the amount secured is insufficient, another supply may be gotten in the same manner.

166. HONOHONO or MAKOLOKOLO. (*Commelina nudiflora*)

This grass grows most abundantly in swampy places. The leaves are oblong in shape. It is largely used as a covering for underground oven.

The value of this grass as a remedy is for purifying the blood. The preparation is as follows:

Chop to small bits enough of the grass to fill about a quart; take four pieces of the bark of the *Bobea* spp.; four pieces of the "koa-ia" bark; a similar amount of the *Aleurites moluccana* bark; a like amount of the mountain apple bark; four *Punex gigauteus* roots; four bulbs of the *Curcuma louza;* four *Morinda citrifolia* fruits that are partly ripe; a teaspoonful and a half of the juice of the red sugar-cane. Have all these materials thoroughly pounded each by itself and then mix them together in a container. Add to the mixture about a quart and a half of water and mix the entire contents thoroughly. Put into the container about twelve red-hot stones with which to cook the whole thing. After being cooked, the container is put where the content would cool off and then the liquid is strained with the fibers of the *Cyperus laevigata* and put into another container. The patient takes a mouthful of this liquid for a single dose three times a day. Salty foods should be avoided at all times.

167. MA-KO-U. (*Peuceda num sandwicense*)

The plant is not very large and it grows along the beach. The leaves are like the palm of the hand and the flowers are long. The bark is smooth and the juice from it is somewhat slimy. The odor is very fragrant and agreeable to the taste. For the expectant mother, it is good to take, for the slimy substance has a healthy effect on the growing life. The mother may begin eating the bark when the developing life is about four months old; and, when it is six months old, the amount is increased to four pieces at a time. She continues to consume this amount until the child is delivered.

From the time the child is born and for twenty days after, the mother may suspend eating the bark but after that period she again resumes the use of it until the child is one year old, when the remedy is fed to him directly. This remedy acts as a mild laxative and it helps to keep the bowels soft.

168. MAMAKI. (*Pipturus* spp.)

This tree grows near the rocky areas of mountains and cliffs. The wood is very hard and for this reason it is largely used for making clubs with which to beat the tapa. The meat of the seeds of this tree is frequently used for the cure of the general debility of the body, both of adults and of children. The preparation is as follows:

For an expectant mother, she begins eating the meat of four "mamaki" seeds when the child is five months old. She continues consuming this amount until the child is seven months old. After this, she takes eight seeds at a time and continues taking this amount until the child is born. After delivering the child, the mother may rest for ten days. After this the mother takes two seeds and feeds the child directly. When the child is months after birth, it may be trained to eat the seeds itself. When this is accomplished, the child is given eight seeds at a time. When it is one year old, the remedy may be changed.

169. WAUKE or WAUKE-MALULO. (*Touchardia latifolia*)

This plant grows near the mountains and can be grown when cultivated. The bark is somewhat grayish. The fiber from this plant is very tough and is frequently made into fishing lines or ropes. The young shoots of this plant are used for the cure of bodily ailments or weaknesses. This is the preparation:

For a child ten days old, four young shoots are chewed and given to it. This is continued until the child is one month old. After this, the child is given eight young shoots and this is continued until he is four months old. From four to eight months, he is given twelve young shoots; and from this age to one year he is given sixteen young shoots. This is the last of this kind of treatment. After this, and until the child is two years old, he is given *Peperomia* spp. treatment. Two doses are taken each day.

For adults, sixteen young shoots may be consumed for a single dose, followed by the eating of a piece of matured cocoanut and a piece of baked taro. Water may be taken immediately after. If necessary, laxative may be taken; and, for this purpose, the "wauke" itself may be used. This is the preparation:

The slimy substance of the plant is scraped off until two tablespoonsful are secured and this is emptied into about a pint of water mixed with a tablespoonful of the milk of the *Euphobia multiformis*. This, again, is mixed with two tablespoonsful of the juice of a young watermelon thoroughly baked. The liquid obtained from such a mixture is then strained with the fibers of the *Cyperus laevigata*. The patient then drinks the whole thing at once, followed by the eating of a banana. Should the remedy prove too laxative, this effect may be stopped by taking a drink of water.

The following are additions from Mr. D. K. Kaaiakamanu. These are not alphabetically arranged

MOKUHALII. (No scientific name given.)

This plant, having thin leaves of grayish color, grows on aged "koa" trees. The tea from this plant is good for a cold and fever. It is also good for a sweat-bath.

NAU-NAU. (No scientific name.)

This plant is soft and is found everywhere. This is very effective for broken bones.

NAU-PAKA. (*Scaevolo frutescens*)

This plant grows along the beach. The bark of the roots is good for cuts when thoroughly pounded and mixed with salt. It is also good for skin diseases.

NIOI.

This plant has very hard wood and grows on Mauna Loa, Molokai. Its other name is "kauila." This plant, as a remedy, is good for skin diseases, scrofulous sores, asthma and bad blood. The wood is scraped into a bowl of *Piper methysticum* drink and taken every night.

NIOI. (*Coprosma* sp.)

The leaves, wood and, in fact, the entire plant, is good to dry and to keep on hand. When needed, it can be easily gotten. The application of it, however, should be under the direction of a medicine man, "kahuna."

MANAWANAWA. (*Vitex trifolia* var. *unifoliolata*)

This plant grows along the beach. The leaves are somewhat round, and fragrant. The other name for it is "na-maka-o-kahai." The leaves are eaten with dried cocoanut. The tea from the leaves and wood thoroughly pounded makes a good bath.

MANAKO. (Mango.)

The leaves are good for tea.

MANENA. (*Pelea cinerea*)

The bark of this tree is whitish and its juice very bitter. As a remedy it is good for venereal diseases.

NIOI. .(Common chili pepper.)

When the seeds are pounded together with salt, it makes good remedy for pains in the back, for swollen feet and for rheumatism.

NIU. (*Cocos nucifera*)

The young shoot of the cocoanut is good for deep cuts.

The ashes of the dried meat of the cocoanut is good for the general debility of the body.

The young meat of the cocoanut is good for the brain. It is applied as rub.

The oil from the shell of the cocoanut is a good rub also.

The smoke from the shell is good for swollen womb.

NONI. (*Morinda citrifolia*)

This tree grows everywhere. The leaves are good for medicine.

The young fruit is good for broken bones and for deep cuts, when thoroughly pounded with salt. The juice from cooked fruit is equally effective. The ripe fruit is specially good when mixed with the other remedies.

NUHOLANI. (Eucalyptus.)

The leaves of this tree are used for sweat bath in fever cases.

The oil is good for rubbing over sores, sprains, backaches and rheumatic pain. It is also good for cuts.

PA-U-O-HIIAKA. (*Jacqemontia sandwicensis*)

This is a creeping plant like the *Impomea dissecta*. As a remedy, this is good for babies having general weakness of the body. It is also good for cuts. This is mixed with taro leaves and pounded with salt. When the leaves and stems are dried, they make good tea. They are also eaten with dried cocoanut.

PAKA. (*Nicotiana tabacum* and *N. glauca*)

This is common tobacco. This is very effective for removing the pus of scrofulous sores or boils. It is also good for sores of all kinds. The smoke is good for cuts.

PA-LA-A. (*Odonto-glossum chineusis*)

This fern is hardy and has spotted leaves. This makes good tea and its use with the *Campylotheca* tea and other remedies is for softening the bowels, and for destroying constipation.

PA-LA-PA-LA-I. (*Microlepia strigosa*)

This is the mountain fern and is used for the cure of insanity.

PA-NI-NI. (*Opuntia tuna.* Cactus.)

The slimy juice from its large and prickly leaves is good for constipation and for an expectant mother. The roots have equal value.

PA-WALE. (*Punex gigauteus*)

This remedy is good for purifying the blood. It is also good for leprosy, consumption, heart disease and for the general weakness of the body. It is used for conditioning the mother for pregnancy.

PI-LI-KAI. (*Argyreia tiliaefolia*)

This vine grows along the beach. It has whitish leaves and the seeds are black. The color of the meat of the seeds is yellowish. This makes a very good laxative.

PO-HUE-HUE. (*Impomea pes-caprae*)

This vine grows along the beach. It is good for the expectant mother.

PO-HE-PO-HE.   (*Hydrogotyle poltata*)

This plant grows in ditches, along the banks of taro-patches, and in fish-ponds. The leaves are round with long stems. This remedy is good for mixing with the other remedies. It is good for the general weakness of the body, lung troubles and diseases of the sexual organs.

WI-LI-WI-LI.   (*Erythrina monosperma*)

This tree grows in dry places and in stony or rocky ground. When dried, the wood becomes very light. The flowers are very effective for venereal diseases. The tea from it is very helpful for diseases of the sexual organs. The bark is pounded and mixed with spring water and taken as a drink. When mixed with the chili pepper and with the *Pelea cinerea* and then taken with the *Piper methysticum*, it becomes a very strong dose. It is taken every evening. The *Impomea dissecta* should be taken every morning.